TOTAL
FITNESS

Kenneth L. Jones
Louis W. Shainberg
Curtis O. Byer

MT. SAN ANTONIO COLLEGE

CANFIELD PRESS
SAN FRANCISCO

A Department of
Harper & Row, Publishers, Inc.

TOTAL FITNESS

International Standard Book Number 0-06-384362-5

LIBRARY OF CONGRESS CATALOG CARD NUMBER: 72-75671

72   73   74   10   9   8   7   6   5   4   3   2   1

RA
776
J77 /18,793

CONTENTS

PREFACE

One of the critical issues confronting humans today is their use of leisure time. Too often, people spend such time in front of television sets or as members of audiences watching others perform. Modern technology also inhibits physical activity; machines perform much of the work once done by human muscles. Automobiles, for example, limit the opportunities people have for obtaining exercise naturally, in the course of performing other activities. Today, then, many people lead sedentary lives; and millions of them have become concerned with their physical fitness and its deterioration.

Physical deterioration is the major underlying cause of death in the United States. In the last one hundred years life expectancy has almost doubled. However, many people spend their last years prisoners of diseases such as emphysema, heart attack, stroke, and senility. It is important to reverse this trend toward physical deterioration, especially if life expectancy continues to increase. To do this, individuals must spend part of their leisure time in activities which provide adequate exercise. A person who is physically fit can avoid debilitating diseases for many more years than can someone who is not fit.

There are a number of books devoted to physical fitness. In the majority, a distinction is made between muscular fitness and cardiovascular fitness. Unfortunately, in most of these books the principles of the two types of fitness are not interrelated.

Books emphasizing muscular fitness are concerned with exercises, weight training, or calisthenics which build muscle tissue. The average person should have an adequate physique but should not be so overdeveloped that he exceeds the weight on the ideal weight table. Excess weight, even from muscle tissue, can be dangerous to the cardiovascular system late in life.

Books emphasizing cardiovascular fitness usually do not mention the necessity for developing muscular strength before performing the recommended physical activities. Often, they recommend that a person perform a series of activities and assess his fitness by his performance. Such tests may easily cause undue fatigue and may, therefore, be dangerous for people with hidden heart and circulatory diseases.

In *Total Fitness* the authors discuss both muscular and cardiovascular fitness and coordinate them into a total program which should help an individual choose the best aspects of each. The program will also help him prepare himself to perform in activity programs throughout life, for a regular physical fitness program should be devoted to maintaining the body in the condition needed to perform sports such as skiing, tennis, and bicycling.

Motivation is the key to total fitness. If a person is to maintain a regular activity program throughout life, he must start early and form the necessary habits. Today, there are too many "weekend athletes" who die of heart attacks because they have not participated in regular programs throughout the week.

K.L.J.
L.W.S.
C.O.B.

Chapter 1

THE MEANING OF PHYSICAL FITNESS

Fitness, according to Dr. Roger Bannister (the first person to run the mile in four minutes), is one of the most misused words in the English language. It can mean anything from "that feeling of pleasure which a person experiences when he stands by an open window early in the morning to—for those with vested interests—some recommendation that we ought to drink more milk or beer." Yet, fitness does have specific implications and important consequences for health.

TOTAL FITNESS

Fitness implies the ability to function at an optimum level of efficiency in all daily living. Fitness, then, means *total fitness*. The concept of total fitness encompasses the whole philosophy of health: the social, emotional, and physical condition of the individual. Total fitness involves intellectual, emotional, and social, as well as physical, conditioning. A totally fit individual has the strength, speed, agility, endurance, and social and emotional adjustments appropriate to his age.

A standard definition of fitness and a standard way of measuring a person's degree of fitness have eluded both physical educators and physiologists for years. Physical educators tend to use performance tests of various skills as a measurement of fitness. Specific performance tests can serve as indicators of the underlying fitness of a part or all of the body, but most measure only one component of total fitness. No single test that measures all aspects of fitness has been devised. Existing programs and tests often measure muscular fitness, or *athletic ability:* strength, speed, and agility. According to these criteria of fitness, an athlete is a person who is physically fit and makes maximum use of his training.

In addition to mobility and muscular strength, physiologists list other important criteria for fitness. Although performance tests are reliable indicators of athletic ability, the most pertinent indicator of physiological fitness is *aerobic capacity* (maximum oxygen consumption).

All body actions require energy. How the body acquires and uses energy is explained in Chapter 3. Very simply, however, energy is produced when the body breaks down foods (carbohydrates, fats, and proteins) in the presence of oxygen. Food and oxygen combine chemically to produce energy. The body can store food, but it cannot store oxygen. If more than a needed amount of food is eaten, the body uses what it needs and stores the rest for later. Since they cannot store oxygen, humans must breathe in and out every moment of their lives to keep the supply coming in. If an individual's oxygen supply is suddenly cut off, the oxygen stored in the body does not last more than a few minutes. The brain, the heart, and all other body tissues cease to function, and the individual dies.

Obtaining oxygen is not a problem; it is breathed in from the air as it is needed. There is a problem, however, in circulating enough oxygen to the parts of the body where food is burned so that the food and oxygen can combine to produce energy. Because people need a constant supply of oxygen to all parts of the body, physiologists have begun to consider a person's aerobic capacity (his maximum oxygen intake and consumption) as the indicator of his physiological fitness or "functioning fitness." A person with a satisfactory aerobic capacity should have the ability to engage in prolonged physical activity (tennis, swimming, bicycling, etc.) without undue fatigue.

Most people produce enough energy to perform ordinary daily activities, that is, to walk, talk, think, and study. However, as activities become more vigorous, they eventually reach their maximum performance, or maximum oxygen consumption. This spread—the difference between minimum energy requirements and maximum capacity—is the physiological measure of fitness. The most physically fit persons have the greatest spread; the least fit have the least spread. In some people the minimum energy requirement and maximum capacity are almost identical. Such physiological measurements of the body systems seem to provide an accurate means of determining fitness.

Another indicator of fitness is *body composition.* The interdependence between nutrition and physical activity is shown by the relative proportion of lean body mass and fat. Throughout life, a relatively high ratio of lean body mass and fat is maintained by individuals who undergo regular physical activity. Such individuals also have satisfactory aerobic capacities, for oxygen is easily circulated to all parts of the body.

THREE CATEGORIES OF FITNESS

Many individuals may be classified into one of three physical fitness categories.

Passive Fitness

The nonexerciser belongs to the category of passive fitness. This individual makes no effort to keep his body fit. He does only what he has to during his daily routine. There is nothing physically wrong with him—not yet—nor is there anything really right with him. If he is lucky, he may remain in this condition for years. However, his body is essentially deteriorating. It will continue to deteriorate unless he increases his physical activity.

Muscular Fitness

Individuals who overemphasize isometrics or isotonics represent muscular fitness. These people have the right motives but the wrong approach. Such individuals subscribe to the myth that muscular strength is equivalent to overall fitness. The skeletal muscles make up only one system in the body; it is by no means the most important system.

Isometrics and isotonic exercises affect primarily the muscular system; although they have some effect on other body systems, their effects on total fitness are limited. Individuals who have only muscular strength may not have the endurance and agility necessary for total fitness.

Total Fitness

Total fitness is achieved when someone engages in balanced activities which strengthen all body systems, particularly the cardiovascular, respiratory, nervous, and muscular systems. It is important to realize, however, that total fitness is produced by *optimum* intensity and duration of physical activity. The amount and duration of physical activity required is different for every person.

Physical activities should match one's likes and needs. The likelihood that a person will maintain a physical fitness program depends on how interesting it is. If someone is to engage in an activity program for many years, it must capture his interest. Most of the well-publicized physical fitness programs which stress exercises and machines or which involve athletic clubs require great motivation over a long period of time. Individual and dual sports may provide good exercise programs because they are fun. Of course, no one can receive satisfaction from a sport which he is not in condition to perform. Consequently, an individual must choose a general conditioning program which may be easily maintained and which will help him remain in condition to take part in the sports of his choice.

The main goal of this book is to motivate you to participate in an activity program which is interesting, challenging, and of sufficient fun that you will want to continue with it. Such an overall program will improve the condition of your lungs, your cardiovascular system, and the total fitness of your body.

FITNESS PROGRAMS

Our knowledge of maximum limits of human physiological fitness and of performance capacities has come mainly from studies of outstanding adult and adolescent athletes, highly trained for specialized events. If the average person is to increase his aerobic capacity and achieve and maintain a reasonable degree of fitness, he must engage in regular physical activity. Activity causes beneficial changes in the functioning of all internal organs, particularly the heart, lungs, and circulatory system. Of course, it also plays a major role in maintaining good weight control.

Fitness programs can be intelligently planned to meet the physiological fitness and skill performance goals recommended for individuals. The goals will differ from person to person, but all people should take part in some kind of fitness program. This is true for children, as well as for adults.

During a child's pre-school years, the neuromuscular system grows and matures, and locomotor movement patterns begin to be established. At this time, the child should undertake activities which contribute to his strength and agility (coordination). Such activities also aid the development of the physiological processes of the organs and tissues of the body systems. For school children, activities may be planned to achieve specific objectives: the development of muscular strength, endurance, and aerobic capacities. They should also be planned for the development of skill, coordination, and a wide range of motion so that the child develops neuromuscular coordination.

For adults, the development of overall fitness requires regular periods of physical activity coupled with the use of the *overload principle*. In using this principle, an individual gradually increases stress, in terms of such factors as speed, work load, and duration of activity. The intensity of an activity should be as high as possible, based on the individual's tolerance level. An activity should last for at least thirty minutes every other day. If an activity is to be beneficial, heart rate must increase dramatically during the course of the activity. The heart rate of the individual at rest should be increased to about 60 percent of the maximum heart rate. Programs which require large amounts of energy (running, swimming, skiing, etc.) improve aerobic capacity and cardiovascular functioning and reduce fat percentage of the body.

To be fit, a person must be in condition. Overall fitness is endurance fitness, or working capacity (the ability to do such prolonged work without undue fatigue). It has much to do with the body's overall health—the health of the lungs, the heart, other body organs, and the entire cardiovascular system, as well as the muscles. The American Medical Association's Committee on Exercise and Physical Fitness (1967) defined physical fitness as "the general capacity to adapt and respond favorably to physical effort. The degree of physical fitness depends on the individual's state of health, constitution and present and previous activity." This is actually a statement of total fitness.

SUMMARY

I. Fitness is frequently misused; it may mean anything from a feeling of pleasure to a commercial recommendation.
II. Total Fitness
    A. Total fitness implies the ability to function at an optimum level of efficiency in all daily living. It encompasses the whole philosophy of health:
        1. The social condition of the individual.
        2. The emotional condition.
        3. The physical condition.
    B. A standard definition of fitness and a standard way of measuring it have eluded physical educators and physiologists for years.
    C. Physical educators tend to use performance tests, which measure athletic ability.
    D. Physiologists consider aerobic capacity (maximum oxygen consumption) to be a pertinent indicator of physiological fitness.

     1. All body activities require energy. Energy is produced by breaking down foods in the presence of oxygen. Food and oxygen combine chemically to produce energy.

       a. The body can store food.

       b. Oxygen cannot be stored; people must breathe in and out every moment of their lives.

       c. Oxygen must constantly circulate to all parts of the body.

     2. Because people need a constant supply of oxygen, the aerobic capacity, or the maximum oxygen intake and consumption of a person, is an indicator of overall fitness. The size of the spread between minimum energy requirements and maximum energy requirements and maximum performance (maximum oxygen consumption) indicates the degree of fitness.

  E. Body composition is an indicator of fitness.

     1. There is an interdependence between nutrition and physical activity and the relative proportion of lean body mass and fat.

     2. A relatively high ratio of lean body mass and fat is maintained by physically fit individuals.

III. Three Categories of Fitness

  A. Passive fitness is a category for people who make no effort to keep their bodies fit.

  B. Muscular fitness is a category for people who overemphasize isometrics or calisthenics.

  C. Total fitness is achieved by people who engage in balanced activities which strengthen all body systems.

IV. Fitness Programs

  A. Regular physical activity is required for an individual to achieve and maintain a reasonable degree of fitness. Activity promotes beneficial changes in all body systems and increases aerobic capacity.

  B. Fitness programs can be intelligently planned to meet the physilogical fitness and skill performance goals recommended for individuals.

  C. Overall fitness requires regular periods of physical activity coupled with the overload principle.

     1. Overload principle—there must be a gradual increase in stress, in terms of such factors as the following:

       a. Speed.

       b. Workload.

       c. Duration of activity.

     2. To be fit, a person must be in condition. He must have the ability to do prolonged work without undue fatigue.

QUESTIONS FOR REVIEW

1. What is total fitness? What does the term totally fit imply?
2. Define athlete.
3. Describe the concept of fitness in terms a physical educator might use. Then describe the concept in terms an exercise physiologist might use. Compare and contrast the two descriptions.
4. Design a series of performance tests of various skills which could measure physical fitness. Which systems of the body would these tests tend to measure most frequently?
5. Explain aerobic capacity. Explain in essay form, how aerobic capacity might affect the systems of the body. Which systems would be most affected? Do these systems differ from the ones you named in answer to question 4?
6. Explain the three categories of fitness described in this chapter. Into which category do you fit? Is this the category into which you would like to be classified? If not, design a schedule which, if followed, would permit you to be classified in the desired category. (After answering this question, check Chapters 5 and 6.)

Chapter 2

THE SKELETAL AND MUSCULAR SYSTEMS

The ability to move the body is one of the essential properties of human life. It is a keystone to the ability of a person to adapt to physical conditions around him. Movements also have aesthetic value. There is fascination and mystique in the manner in which a person moves.

All body movements depend upon the activity of muscles in association with specific bones. The skeleton consists of all the bones of the body and the cartilage and ligaments which hold bones together. The skeleton serves three major functions; protection, support, and, in association with the muscles, movement.

THE SKELETAL SYSTEM

The skeleton consists of two subdivisions: the *axial skeleton*, the central axis of the body, and the *appendicular skeleton*, the bones of the shoulders, hips, arms, and legs (Figure 2.1).

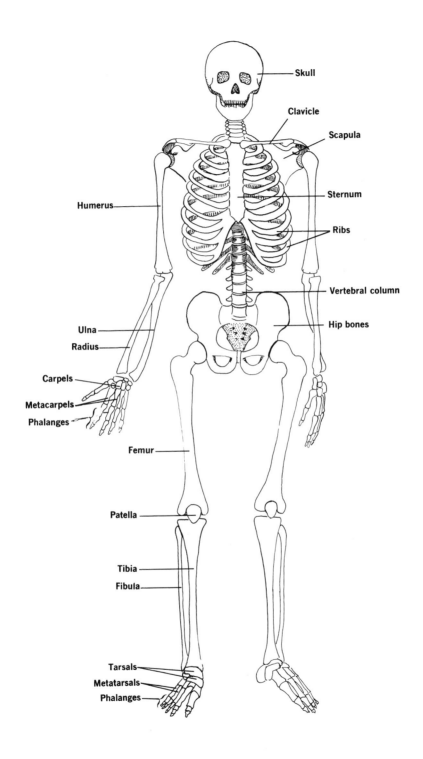

Figure 2.1 Human skeleton, front view.

The bones of the body may be classified into four general types in terms of their shapes: *long bones,* as in arms and legs; *short bones,* as in the wrists and ankles; *flat bones,* as in the skull and chest; and *irregular bones,* as in the vertebral column.

The adult skeleton consists of 206 bones. At birth, however, as many as 270 bones may be identified. The reduced number in the adult results from the union, or fusion, of a number of bones which are separate in the infant.

Axial Skeleton

The axial skeleton consists of the skull, vertebral column, ribs, and breastbone. In the adult this represents eighty bones.

SKULL

The skull (cranium and face) is formed by twenty-nine bones. Many of these are flat and become inseparably joined along jagged edges, or *sutures.* Several bones form the top of the skull: the *frontal bone,* which forms the forehead; the two *parietal bones,* which start at the top and form the two sides of the skull; the *occipital bone,* which forms the back of the skull; the *temporal bones,* found around and

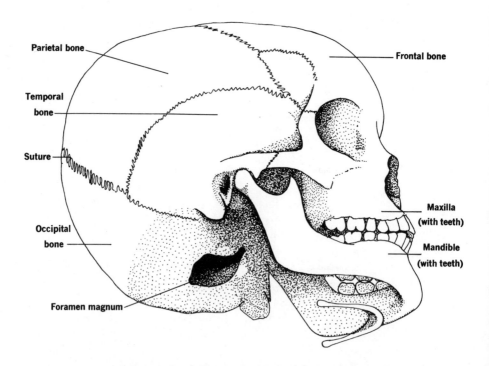

Figure 2.2   Skull, side view (inferior aspect).

above each ear; the *hyoid bone,* and the six small bones *(ossicles)* in the middle ear (Figure 2.2.)

There are many bones making up the face. These vary in shape and size, depending on age, race, sex, and individual differences. They determine the contour of the face.

VERTEBRAL COLUMN

Also known as the backbone, or spinal column, the vertebral column connects the shoulders to the hips and supports the head. In the infant it consists of thirty-three irregular bones. In the adult several of these have fused, reducing the count to twenty-six. The *vertebrae* are constructed with a *body* to support the next vertebra, an *arch* to provide space for the spinal cord, and *processes* (spines) to give muscles something to which they can attach (Figure 2.3). Between every two vertebra is a disk of cartilage (similar to the soft tissue in the end of the nose or earlobe) which helps both to hold the vertebrae together and to cushion them as a person moves.

The vertebral column is divided into five sections. The seven *cervical* vertebrae make up the neck, and the twelve *thoracic* support the ribs. There are five *lumbar* vertebrae in the lower part of the back. There is a single *sacrum,* which connects to the pelvis, and a single *coccyx,* or tailbone.

RIB CAGE

The rib cage consists of twelve pairs of ribs. These are held together in front with a *sternum* (breastbone), which you can feel as you tap the middle of your chest.

Appendicular Skeleton

The appendicular skeleton consists of the two arms, the two legs, the shoulder bones (pectoral girdle), and the hipbones (pelvic girdle). It is made up of 126 bones.

THE ARMS AND PECTORAL GIRDLE

As seen in Figure 2.1, there is a ring of bones making up the shoulders. This ring is known as the *pectoral girdle,* and it supports the arms. This girdle consists of the two collarbones *(clavicles),* which can be felt on the front of the shoulder, and the two shoulder blades *(scapulae),* which are deeply embedded in muscle on the back of the shoulders. The breastbone connects the two collarbones in the front.

Suspended from the ends of the shoulders are the arms. The upper arm *(humerus)* extends to the elbow. The lower arm consists of two bones. These are in a side-by-side position when the arm is held with the palm of the hand up. In this position the lower arm bone on the thumb side is the *radius;* and the one on the little finger side is the *ulna.*

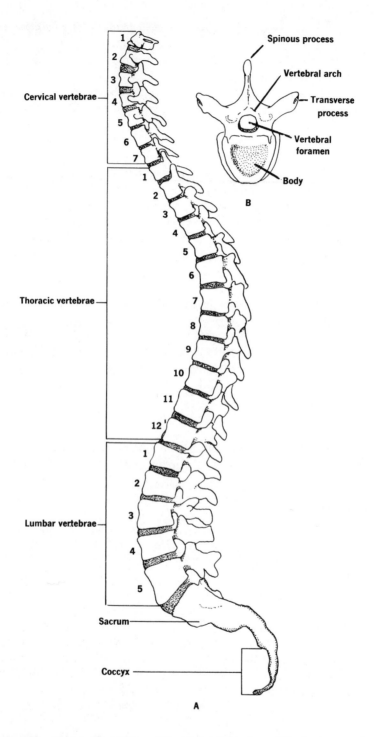

Cervical vertebrae

Thoracic vertebrae

Lumbar vertebrae

Sacrum

Coccyx

Spinous process

Vertebral arch

Transverse process

Vertebral foramen

Body

B

A

Figure 2.3 Vertebral column. (A) whole side view. (B) single vertebra, top view.

The wrist is formed by eight small bones, the *carpals*. The hand consists of the *metacarpals*, five small bones embedded in the muscle of the palm, and the *phalanges*, the three bones in each finger and the two bones in the thumb.

THE LEGS AND PELVIC GIRDLE

The *pelvic girdle* is made of two hipbones, one on each side of the body. They are connected to the sacrum in the back and to each other in the front. Each hipbone is actually made up of three bones which have fused together.

The legs connect to the pelvic girdle. The upper leg, or thigh-bone (*femur*), extends to the knee. This is the longest and heaviest bone of the body. Protecting the knee is the kneecap *(patella)*, which you can easily feel. The lower leg, or shank, consists of two bones. The shin-bone *(tibia)* is the bone easily felt on the front of the lower leg. The *fibula* is smaller and deeply embedded in muscle. The ankle of the foot is made up of seven tarsals. One of these forms the heel of the foot. The palm, or body of the foot, consists of five metatarsals. The big toe is made up of two phalanges, and toes two through five are each constructed of three phalanges. In order to support the weight of the body, the tarsals and metatarsals are formed into strong arches. Ligaments, tendons, and muscles help to maintain the arches.

Bones and Exercise

Bones are very much alive. The shape and composition of bones change with age. In young children bones tend to be elastic. As a person matures his bones become heavier and tougher. In old age there is a reduction in the amount of living matter in bones, and they become considerably lighter and more fragile.

Bones also adapt their structure to the sorts of stress placed on them. Stress placed on the skeletal muscles is transmitted to the bones. Strain applied to the leg bones over a long period of time causes them to become thicker. The bones of athletes are considerably thicker and heavier than those of nonathletes. When a particular part of a bone is subjected to continuing stress, that part becomes thicker. It also becomes rougher at the points of muscle attachment due to muscular stress, greatly strengthening the attachment of the muscles to the bone. The shape and thickness of bones reflect the attachment of ligaments and muscle tendons and the sorts of strains those muscles have exerted on the bones.

Joints

The region where one bone meets another is called a *joint*. Some joints are movable while others are not. There are three major kinds of joints in the body:

1. *No Movement*. Bone tissue forms between some joints,

solidly fusing them together. The sacrum in the vertebral column was once five individual bones. The coccyx was once four individual bones. The cranial and facial bones interlock along the sutures to form immovable joints.

2. *Slight Movement.* Some joints are held together by fibrous tissue in which there is slight movement. Such fibers hold the vertebrae of the vertebral column together but allow a limited movement in every direction.

3. *Free Movement.* Most joints of the body fall into this category. The adjacent ends of two bones are covered with *cartilage.* Tough connective tissues, or *ligaments,* hold one bone to the other. The joint is encased within a capsule which is filled with a fluid lubricant. This fluid helps to keep the cartilage-covered ends of the bones slightly apart, and it cushions them. It also supplies nutrients to the tissues of the joints and removes wastes. Where pressure is exerted over moving bones, there may also be other small fluid-filled sacs called *bursae.* When these sacs become inflamed, the condition is called *bursitis.*

Freely moving joints may be classified into three main categories: *gliding joints,* as in the wrist and ankle; *hinge joints,* as in the knee or elbow; and *ball-and-socket joints,* as in the hip and the shoulder. An example of each kind of joint may be seen in Figure 2.1.

MUSCLES AND BODY MOVEMENTS

All body movements depend upon the activity of muscles. By definition a *muscle* is an organ made up of bundles of contractile fibers by which movement is brought about. There are three distinct kinds of muscle tissue found in the human body: *skeletal,* which provides the force for the movement of bones; *smooth,* which is found in the walls of the digestive tract and blood vessels; and *cardiac,* which is found only in the heart. In this book we will be concerned primarily with skeletal muscles.

Since the movement of bones is controlled by muscles, muscles must be firmly attached to the bones. Muscles attach indirectly to bones by *tendons* (Figure 2.4). The surfaces of bones where tendons attach are usually roughened. This can be easily seen by looking at an arm or a leg of a human skeleton.

Skeletal muscles generally attach to two different bones. Such muscles have an attachment end *(origin)* and a movement end *(insertion),* as shown in Figure 2.4. Such a muscle might be compared to a rope used to pull water skiers. The end of the rope anchored to the boat would be the origin, and the action end which the water skier holds (and which moves freely) would be the insertion.

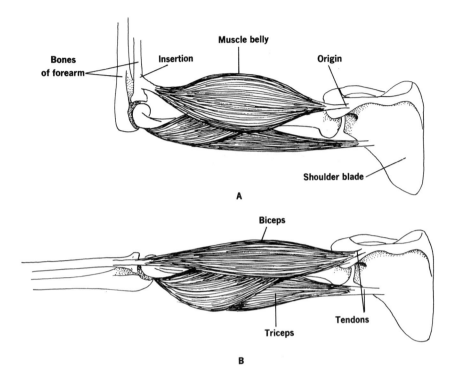

Figure 2.4 Muscles showing insertion and origin. Upper arm. (A) Bended arm. (B) Extended arm.

Structure of Skeletal Muscles

People without technical training can observe that several types of tissue are present in skeletal muscle. Almost everyone has eaten beefsteak. It is easy to see that this steak contains at least three kinds of tissue. The fatty tissue is merely a reservoir for the storage of fat. The tough connective tissue, however, is very important. It surrounds the muscle fibers, bundling the muscle tissues tightly together. The connective tissue also joins with the tendon to connect the muscle securely to the bone so that movement can occur.

All skeletal muscles consist of many muscle fibers. The larger the muscle, the more fibers it contains. Fibers run parallel to the length, or long axis, of the muscle. When fibers contract, the muscle contracts.

Each muscle fiber is encased by connective tissue, in the way that a sausage is enclosed inside its covering. Bundles of such fibers are, in turn, enclosed by connective tissue. Furthermore, groups of muscle-fiber bundles are wrapped together by an outer connective tissue. Scattered throughout the connective tissue are nerves and blood vessels which supply the muscle fibers with nutrients and transmit messages which tell the muscles when to contract. The bundles of fibers are shown in the cross section of a skeletal muscle in Figure 2.5.

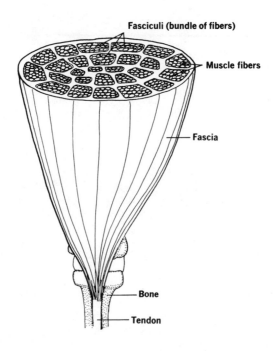

Figure 2.5   Section of a skeletal muscle showing muscle fibers.

Body Movements

A muscle contracts because each muscle fiber composing it becomes "excited." Anything which brings about this excitability is called a *stimulus*. If a muscle fiber is excited at one place along its length, the response will travel up or down the entire fiber. Muscle fibers respond to a stimulus by *contracting*. Muscle fibers are normally stimulated by impulses carried to them by nerve cells. Muscle fibers can also be stimulated with artificial stimuli, such as electric current (commonly used in biology laboratories).

Any stimulus strong enough to cause a response in a muscle fiber will cause it to produce a maximum contraction, regardless of the strength of the stimulus. This is called the *all-or-none law*. Either a muscle fiber contracts or it doesn't. The intensity of contraction in the whole muscle depends upon how many muscle fibers are made to contract at one time.

Skeletal muscles contract quickly and relax promptly. When a stimulus arrives at the muscle, the intensity of the contraction (the number of fibers made to contract) is influenced by several factors: the strength of the stimulus reaching the muscle, the speed with which the stimulus is applied, the length of time the stimulus lasts, the weight or tension of the work load to be done, and the temperature of the body.

In humans optimum working conditions for muscles seem to be a normal body temperature of about 98.6°F., a moderate weight load, and stimuli of moderate duration.

When a muscle is stimulated to contract many times in succession, the contractions become more intense until they reach a point of maximum intensity. Thus, a "staircase" effect is created. If a second stimulus arrives while a muscle is at the peak of contraction, a maximum contraction will reoccur. This is called *summation of contractions*. If successive stimuli arrive so rapidly that each occurs before the muscle can relax from the preceding stimulus, the muscle will maintain a state of steady contraction, or *tetanus*. All voluntary acts of the body can be carried out because of tetanic contractions of the body muscles. Tetanic contractions permit people to hold their bodies erect, and to carry loads, for example. Posture is the result of a state of tetanus.

Muscle tone (tonus) exists when partial contraction (involving a small number of fibers) is maintained in a muscle. Muscle tone allows posture to be maintained for long periods of time with little or no fatigue. Fatigue is avoided mainly by different groups of muscle fibers contracting in relays; this gives muscle groups alternating periods of rest and activity. In humans the greatest degree of tone is seen in the neck and back muscles. In an unconscious person the body collapses because these muscles are completely relaxed. During periods of sleep, tone is at a minimum. Tone is also exhibited in the walls of small arteries (maintaining blood pressure) and in the walls of the stomach and intestine (assuring the movement of materials through the digestive tract).

If a person exercises intensely, his muscles undergo a period of prolonged contractions. If the muscles are continuously stimulated over a long period of time, they do not have an opportunity to dispose of waste materials, such as carbon dioxide, and to replace oxygen and nutrients. Unless rested, the muscles will eventually suffer an oxygen deficiency and a buildup of carbon dioxide and other wastes. Then they will refuse to respond. The inability of a muscle to contract is called *muscle fatigue*.

When exercise is moderate, the body can eliminate wastes easily. Furthermore, exercise is beneficial to the body because it changes conditions for all cells. Fresh blood is brought in, and accumulated wastes are removed. Exercise increases the size, strength, and tone of muscle fibers. It increases the efficiency of muscle cells and the ability of the body to avoid fatigue.

Although exercise is desirable, use of fatigued muscles may be injurious if the energy supply to the muscle cells becomes too low. Usually, however, the sensation of fatigue protects people from exercising to extremes.

KINDS OF SKELETAL MUSCLES

Skeletal muscles constitute the "red flesh" of the body and account for 42 percent of the male's weight and 36 percent of the female's weight. There are over 400 skeletal muscles in the human body (Figures 2.6 and 2.7). Although no attempt will be made to discuss all of them, the muscles important in exercise will be discussed briefly. Then when you are performing an exercise, you can find the appropriate muscle on your body and determine whether the exercise is actually causing the muscle group to contract.

Muscles of the Head and Neck

These muscles are concerned with mastication (chewing), facial expression, and movement of the head.

The two most significant muscles, for our purposes, are found in the neck. The *sternocleidomastoid,* as the name suggests, is attached to the sternum (breastbone), the clavicle (collarbone), and the mastoid process of the skull. This muscle pulls the head lower toward the shoulder. The pair of sternocleidomastoids, one on either side of the head, helps to keep the head erect.

The *platysma* (meaning "flat piece") arises from the skin of the chest, extends over the front of the neck, and inserts on the lower edge of the lower jaw. It pulls the corners of the mouth and the lower lip downward. When contracted, it can stretch the skin of the neck.

Muscles of the Back and Thorax

The muscle highest on the back is the *trapezius.* This is a large triangular muscle which arises on the back of the skull, fans down the back of the neck, and inserts into the shoulder bones. It can either raise or lower the shoulder. If the shoulder is fixed, it can pull the head backward. The trapezius is important in maintaining posture.

The *latissimus dorsi* is a very large, flat, triangular muscle which covers the lower part of the back. It arises from the lower thoracic and lumbar vertebrae, and the sacrum. It sweeps upward and inserts on the humerus (upper arm bone). Upon contraction, it pulls the arm and shoulder backward and rotates the arm inward. It may show very well on a muscular male (Figure 2.7).

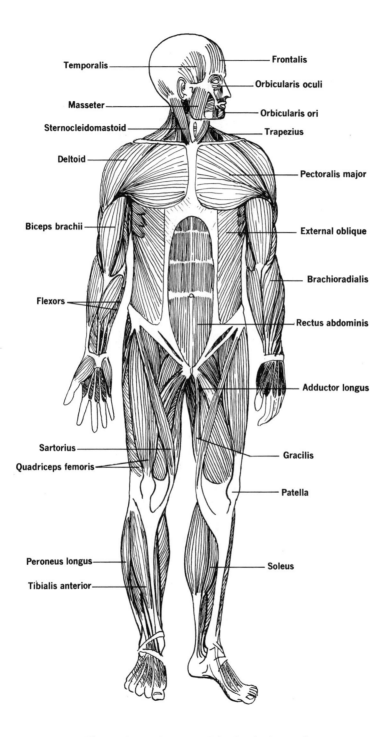

Figure 2.6 Muscles of the body, front view.

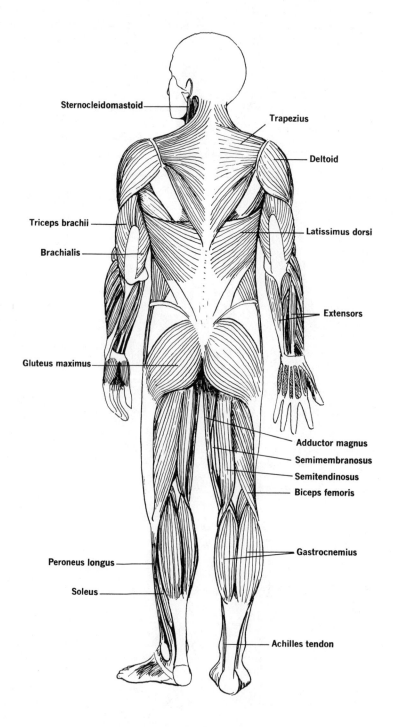

Figure 2.7 Muscles of the body, back view.

There are two *pectoralis major* muscles. Each is a large triangular muscle covering the upper front part of the chest. Each originates along the entire clavicle and the sternum and inserts onto the upper humerus. These important muscles assist in pulling the arms down toward the chest. They also draw the arms across the chest while rotating them inward. The pectoralis majors are often well developed in swimmers.

The *pectoralis minor* is a small muscle located underneath each pectoralis major and entirely covered by it. This muscle arises on the upper margins of the third, fourth, and fifth ribs and inserts onto the upper tips of the scapula (shoulder blade). It draws the shoulders downward when it contracts.

Muscles of the Upper Extremities

The *deltoid* muscles form the muscular caps of each shoulder. Arising on the scapula and clavicle, each deltoid continues down over the shoulder and inserts into the humerus. It is the chief muscle for moving the arm away from the body.

THE UPPER ARM

The *biceps branchii* is often called the biceps. It is the large muscle on the front of the humerus which may bulge conspicuously in a well-developed person (Figure 2.6). The muscle arises at two different locations on the scapula (has two heads, or biceps) and inserts onto the radius of the lower arm. This muscle pulls the arm forward while holding it close to the body and is, therefore, important in the lifting of heavy objects.

The *triceps branchii,* or triceps, arises from three heads, two from the humerus and one from the scapula, and inserts on the ulna of the lower arm. It is sometimes referred to as "the boxer's muscle" since it is the major muscle for straightening the elbow. It opposes the action of the biceps; the biceps bends the elbow, and the triceps straightens it.

Muscles of the Abdomen

Contraction of the abdominal muscles assists in such diverse actions as expiration of air (by forcing the diaphragm up), defecation, childbirth, urination, and maintenance of pressure in the abdomen.

The fibers of the *interior abdominal muscles* run vertically in a belt along the front center of the abdomen. Of these muscles, the primary one is the *rectus abdominis.* These support the internal organs and pull the body forward when contracted.

There are several *posterior abdominal muscles (spinal erectors)* which lie beneath the latissimus dorsi and other muscles of the back. They help to maintain posture, and they prevent people from falling backward when standing.

Muscles of the Lower Extremities

THE HIP AND BUTTOCK

The *gluteus maximus* is the heaviest muscle of the body and forms most of the buttock. Arising from the lower vertebrae and pelvic girdle, it inserts on the femur (thighbone). This muscle helps a person stand erect and is important in walking and running. The buttock is also made up of two smaller muscles, the *gluteus medius and the gluteus minimus.* These muscles help to rotate the femur inward.

On the front of the thigh is the *quadriceps femoris,* a muscle made up of four parts. This muscle arises on the femur and extends to the tibia of the lower leg. The patella (kneecap) is embedded in the tendon which connects this muscle to the lower leg. The quadriceps femoris is the chief straightener (extensor) of the lower leg. It extends the knee when, for example, someone kicks a football. "Charley-horse," the term used to indicate spasm, soreness, and stiffness in a muscle, is most frequently used in relation to this muscle.

The *sartorius* is a long, narrow muscle which begins on the edge of the hipbone, winds downward and inward across the entire thigh, and ends up on the inner side of the lower leg. It is used chiefly in crossing the legs. Because tailors once sat in a cross-legged position, the sartorius is sometimes called "the tailor's muscle."

The *biceps femoris* is a two-headed muscle which arises on the femur and ilium and inserts on the lower leg. The biceps femoris, *semitendinosus,* and *semimembranosus* muscles make up the hamstring muscles. (Butchers used to use the tendons from these muscles of pigs to hang up hams.) These muscles serve chiefly to bend the knee.

The *adductor muscles* extend from the pubic bone (located in front of the body between the legs) to the femur. The word "adduct" means "bring together." Consequently, these muscles bring a person's legs together when he is lying on his back with his legs spread apart.

THE LEG

The *gastrocnemius* is the chief muscle of the calf of the leg and forms its outer curvature (Figure 2.7). The word element *gastr-* means "belly." The gastrocnemius arises near the lower end of the femur and ends near the heel in a prominent cord on the back of the lower leg. The cord, called the *Achilles tendon,* is the largest tendon of the body; it attaches to the heel bone. The gastrocnemius, sometimes called "the toe dancer's muscle," enables a person to rise on the balls of his feet and on his toes; it also helps bend the knee joint. The gastrocnemius of the frog is commonly used for laboratory experiments with muscle.

The *tibialis anterior* muscle arises on the upper part of the tibia and continues across the front of the leg to the inside of the anklebones. It is used to turn the sole of the foot inward and to raise the rest of the foot off the ground when one wants to walk on his heels.

SUMMARY

  I. The Skeletal System

    A. Composed of all the bones of the body and the cartilage and ligaments which hold bones together. The skeleton serves three major functions: protection, support, and in association with the muscles, movement.

    B. Parts

      1. Axial skeleton—the central axis of the body.

      2. Appendicular skeleton—the bones of the shoulders, hips, arms, and legs.

    C. Bones of the skeleton may be classified into four general types in terms of their shapes:

      1. Long bones, as in the arms and the legs.

      2. Short bones, as in the wrists and the ankles.

      3. Flat bones, as in the skull and the chest.

      4. Irregular bones, as in the vertebral column.

    D. At birth, an infant may have as many as 270 bones. An adult has only 206 separate bones.

    E. Axial Skeleton

      1. Skull (formed by twenty-nine bones).

      2. Vertebral column (formed by thirty-three irregular bones).

      3. Rib cage (twelve pairs of ribs held together in front by the sternum, or breastbone).

    F. Appendicular Skeleton

      1. The arms and the pectoral girdle (the ring of bones making up the shoulders).

        a. Bones in the pectoral girdle: clavicles (collarbones) and shoulder blades (scapulae).

        b. Bones in the arm: the humerus (upper arm), the radius and ulna (lower arm), carpals, metacarpals, and phalanges.

      2. The legs and the pelvic girdle

        a. Bones in the pelvic girdle: two hipbones connected to *sacrum* in the back and to each other in the front.

        b. Bones in the legs; the femur (thighbone), the tibia and fibula (lower leg), tarsals, metatarsals, and phalanges.

G. Bones and Exercise
1. Bones are alive.
2. The shape and composition of bones change with age.
3. Bones adapt their structure to the kinds of stress they encounter.
H. Joints
1. The region where one bone meets another is called a joint.
2. Three major kinds of joints in the body:
a. No Movement
b. Slight Movement
c. Free Movement (gliding joints, hinge joints, and ball-and-socket joints)
II. Muscles and Body Movements
A. By definition a muscle is an organ made up of bundles of contractile fibers by which movement is brought about.
B. There are three kinds of muscle tissue in the body:
1. Skeletal Muscle
2. Smooth Muscle
3. Cardiac Muscle
C. Muscles attach indirectly to bones by tendons.
D. Skeletal muscles generally attach to two different bones. Such muscles have an attachment end (origin) and a movement end (insertion).
E. Skeletal muscles consist of many muscle fibers wrapped together by connective tissue into bundles.
F. A muscle contracts because the muscle fibers become "excited" by a stimulus.
G. The intensity of contraction in reaction to a stimulus depends upon several factors:
1. The strength of the stimulus.
2. The speed with which the stimulus is applied.
3. The length of time the stimulus lasts.
4. The weight, or tension, of the load of work to be done.
5. The temperature of the body.
H. Any stimulus strong enough to cause a muscle response produces a maximum contraction (the all-or-none law).
I. Muscle tone (tonus) exists when a steady, partial contraction is maintained in a muscle. Muscle tone allows posture to be maintained for long periods of time with little or no fatigue.
J. Summation of Contractions and Tetanus
1. If a muscle contracts many times in succession, the contractions become more intense (the "staircase" effect). If a second stimulus arrives while a muscle is at the peak of contraction, a maximum contraction will reoccur. This is called summation of contractions.

2. If successive stimuli arrive in such rapid succession that each occurs before the muscle can relax, the muscle will maintain a state of steady contraction, or tetanus.
   a. All voluntary acts of the body are carried out because of tetanic contractions of body muscles.
   b. Posture is the result of tetanus.
K. Fatigue (the inability of a muscle to contract)
   1. Fatigue is caused by overstimulation of a muscle, leading to an oxygen deficiency and a buildup of carbon dioxide and other wastes.
   2. Moderate exercise is beneficial because it helps to bring fresh blood into the body and to eliminate wastes.
III. Kinds of Skeletal Muscles
   A. Muscles of the Head and Neck—concerned mainly with mastication (chewing), facial expression, and movement of the head.
   B. Muscles of the Back and Thorax
      1. Are important in maintaining posture.
      2. Control the shoulder, pull the head backward, and rotate the arm inward.
      3. Pull the arms down across the chest while rotating them inward.
   C. Muscles of the Upper Extremities (the deltoids)
      1. Form the muscular caps of each shoulder.
      2. Move the arms away from the body.
   D. Muscles of the Upper Arm
      1. The biceps branchii pulls the arm forward, while holding it close to the body and is, therefore, important in lifting heavy objects.
      2. The triceps branchii is the major muscle for straightening the elbow.
   E. Muscles of the abdomen assist in expiration of air, defecation, childbirth, urination, and maintenance of pressure in the abdomen.
      1. Anterior Abdominal Muscles
      2. Posterior abdominal muscles help to maintain posture and prevent people from falling backward when standing.
   F. Muscles of the Lower Extremities
      1. Muscles of the Hip and Buttock
         a. Help a person stand erect.
         b. Very important in running and walking.
         c. Flex and extend the legs.
         d. Control the ability to cross the legs.
         e. Bend the knee.
         f. Bring a person's legs together when he is lying on his back with his legs spread apart.

2. Muscles of the Leg
   a. Enable a person to rise on the balls of his feet and on his toes.
   b. Bend the knee joint.
3. Muscles of the Foot
   a. Turn the sole of the foot inward.
   b. Raise the foot off the ground when one wants to walk on his heels.

QUESTIONS FOR REVIEW

1. Describe briefly the different tissues which make up the skeletal system.
2. Explain the functions of the skeleton.
3. Classify the bones into their four basic shapes. Where would you find each of these basic shapes?
4. How many bones are there in the adult skeleton? How many bones are there in the fetal skeleton? What accounts for the difference in the number of bones?
5. What is a joint? Classify the joints of the human body. Give an example of each of the major kinds of joints.
6. What is a muscle? How does a muscle perform its function?
7. Explain the all-or-none law.
8. Explain muscle tone. How is posture maintained? Which muscles are mainly responsible for the posture of the body?

Chapter 3

DIET AND WEIGHT CONTROL

The human body is a very efficient energy-conversion machine. Energy, or the capacity to do work, exists in two basic forms: *potential energy*, the chemical energy of, for example, a sugar cube or a pound of beefsteak; and *kinetic energy*, active forms of energy such as heat, motion, light, and electricity. The human body converts the chemical potential energy of food into kinetic energy in the forms of heat and work (movement).

The unit for expressing the energy content of food is the *large calorie*, or *kilocalorie*. One kilocalorie is the amount of energy required to raise 1 kilogram (2.2 pounds) of water 1° C. Consequently, if an amount of food containing 600 calories was burned and the heat transferred to 1 kilogram of water, the temperature of the water would be raised by 600° C.

ENERGY REQUIREMENTS AND FOOD

The human body uses a considerable amount of energy. All the chemical reactions which require energy make up the *metabolism* of the body. Metabolism includes both those reactions in which food is broken down and energy is released and those in which new substances are produced within the body and energy is stored up.

Such basic functions as breathing, heartbeat, and glandular secretions—"just staying alive"—require energy. An individual's energy expenditure is his *basal metabolic rate* (BMR). It is measured while a person is awake but while he is reclining and completely relaxed. The number of calories required for basal metabolism varies with sex, weight, stature, thyroid level, and hormone production. The basal metabolic rate is highest in childhood and drops gradually throughout life. Therefore, as they get older, people must make a gradual adjustment in eating habits to avoid excess weight gain.

The basal metabolic rate of females is usually lower than that of males. The average adult utilizes some 1500 to 1800 calories per day for his basal metabolism. You may estimate the approximate number of calories needed daily for your basal metabolism by multiplying 1 calorie per hour (24 per day) for each kilogram (2.2 pounds) of body weight. For example, an adult male who is of average stature and weighs 154 pounds (70 kilograms) requires 1680 (24 x 70) calories per day for his basal metabolism.

In addition to the energy needed for basal metabolism, a widely varying quantity of energy is required for everyday activities. An inactive person may utilize as few as 500 additional calories per day, whereas a large, active person (for example, someone doing heavy manual labor) may need several thousand additional calories in a day. Total energy requirements, then, may range from only slightly more than the amount needed for basal metabolism to more than double that amount, depending on the amount of activity a person undertakes.

FOODS

In addition to their obvious function as sources of energy, foods are necessary for several important body functions. Foods supply materials for growth and replacement of worn or damaged cells and for the manufacture of cellular products such as enzymes and hormones. Foods contain materials such as vitamins which are needed in varying amounts for different body functions. Although the hundreds of kinds of food consumed by people may show little outward similarity, foods may be classified into three categories.

Carbohydrates

The carbohydrates consist of sugars and starches. They are the most important sources of energy available. Foods high in carbohydrates include rice, corn, other grains, potatoes, and all sweet foods.

Carbohydrates consisting of combinations of simple sugar units are called *saccharides*. Each simple sugar unit is a *monosaccharide*. The simple sugars are glucose; a form of the same sugar, dextrose; and fructose. Honey and many fruits contain these sugars.

Carbohydrates consisting of two simple sugar units are called *disaccharides*. Examples of disaccharides are sucrose, or common table sugar (cane and beet sugars are identical); maltose, produced by germinating grains; and lactose, found only in milk.

Starches are polysaccharides; that is, they are long chains of simple sugar units (monosaccharides) linked together. The polysaccharide cellulose, although present in most foods which come from plants, cannot be converted into energy by humans, because we lack the digestive enzymes necessary for its breakdown. Cellulose is, however, useful in stimulating intestinal activity, because it adds bulk, or roughage, to the diet.

It matters little whether carbohydrates are consumed in the form of monosaccharides, disaccharides, or polysaccharides, since digestion reduces most of them to their monosaccharide components before they are absorbed into the blood. Monosaccharides other than glucose are further converted by the liver into glucose, the only carbohydrate used as a source of energy by the body's cells.

The primary function of carbohydrates is to supply energy in the body. Each pound of carbohydrates consumed yields 1860 calories of energy. In Table 3.1 the energy values of the basic food groups are compared. If the diet is low in carbohydrates, fats and proteins will be converted into glucose to provide energy. If there is a surplus of carbohydrates in the diet, they are readily converted into human fats and stored in the adipose (the thick, fatty) tissues for possible future use.

Fats

The fats have the highest energy content of any known foods. They yield 4220 calories per pound, providing over twice as much energy as carbohydrates. They also serve as the body's reservoir for the long-term storage of energy. In addition to their use as sources of energy, fats are important to several body functions. Fats are important in the membranes of all cells and in the nerve sheaths. Apparently, humans must have small quantities of fats in their diets if the fat-soluble vitamins are to be absorbed into the blood.

Fats are abundant in foods such as meat, whole milk, cheese, nuts, and olives. Food products such as butter, margarine, oils, and shortenings are almost pure fat. Fortunately, abundant quantities of fats are widely distributed in foods, and fat deficiency is virtually unknown in the United States.

Table 3.1   Energy Values of Basic Food Groups

TYPE OF FOOD	CALORIES PER GRAM	CALORIES PER POUND
Carbohydrates	4.1	1860
Proteins	4.1	1860
Fats	9.3	4220

Proteins

Of the three groups of energy-yielding foods (carbohydrates, fats, and proteins), the proteins are the most essential to life. Proteins are made up of chains of amino acids. Through digestion, proteins are broken down into their component amino acids and are then absorbed into the blood. After they are absorbed into the blood, amino acids are reassembled to form body proteins. Among the twenty common amino acids, only eight are essential and must be present in the human diet. If the remaining twelve amino acids are not obtained through the diet, they can be produced within the body.

Proteins which contain all eight essential amino acids in significant quantities are said to be *of high biological value*. A protein low in one or more of the essential amino acids is said to be of low biological value. Most proteins originating from animal sources are of high value, while many proteins originating from plants are of low value. This is why vegetarians may have difficulty obtaining proper protein nutrition.

Since normal growth and maintenance of the human body are based on amino acids, proteins are of primary importance in the diet. Amino acids may also serve as sources of energy when the diet is high in proteins but low in fats and carbohydrates. Proteins yield 1860 calories per pound, an amount of energy equivalent to that yielded by carbohydrates.

Vitamins

Vitamins are present in minute amounts in natural foods and are essential to the execution of specific chemical reactions. Although vitamins are not sources of energy, they are essential to the proper functioning of the body. The vitamins and their major properties are summarized in Table 3.2.

The recommended daily allowance (RDA) for each vitamin is also shown in Table 3.2. The RDA is the amount required to maintain optimum health. Vitamins may also be rated by minimum daily requirements (MDR), the amount necessary to prevent diseases caused by vitamin deficiency. The U.S. Food and Drug Administration has estab-

lished the MDRs as standards for the labeling of food
tical preparations.

The solubility of a vitamin—whether it is water
—is important because it influences the source of the vitamin,
tion into the body, and its fate within the body. In general, t.
vitamins are more persistent in the body and may have toxic e
consumed in excessive quantities.

The complete absence of a given vitamin from the diet causes
avitaminosis, a condition rare in the United States today. However,
many Americans suffer from *hypovitaminosis* which is caused by a diet
falling below the minimum requirements of one or more vitamins. Such
individuals are not always seriously ill, but they lack the health and
vitality to enjoy life fully.

Minerals

Minerals are consumed as rather simple compounds. Once in
the body, however, they may be incorporated into very complex, vital
body chemicals. Some minerals are vital parts of cells, bones, teeth, and
blood. Others are equally important parts of body products such as
hormones.

Some people now believe that as many as thirteen minerals
are necessary for optimum human health. Essential minerals which are
rarely deficient in the American diet include sodium, potassium, chlor-
ine, coper, sulfur, zinc, manganese, and magnesium. Minerals which
are more likely to be deficient are listed in Table 3.3.

Water

No other chemical compound serves the body in so many
distinct and vital functions as does water. The body weight of humans
is over 65 percent water, and many tissues contain up to 90 percent
water. A human is so dependent on this substance that if his body loses
only 10 percent of its water, he will die.

Water is the medium in which all chemical reactions of metabolism take place. Digestion, absorption, and secretion take place only
in a water medium. Water moistens the surfaces of the lungs so that
diffusion (the movement of oxygen and carbon dioxide) can take
place. Water is vitally important in distributing heat uniformly throughout the body and in eliminating excess heat through evaporation. It is
the vehicle which transports all vital substances throughout the body.
It serves as a cushion for the brain and spinal cord.

A person's daily water requirement depends greatly on the
temperature of his environment (room temperature) and on the
amount of physical activity he engages in. On a cool day a moderately

Table 3.2 Vitamins and Their Major Properties

VITAMIN	RICH SOURCES	PROPERTIES
FAT-SOLUBLE VITAMINS		
Vitamin A	Cheese, green and yellow vegetables, butter, eggs, milk, fish liver oils. Carotene in vegetables converted to vitamin A by liver.	Lost through oxidation during long cooking in open kettle. Overdose possible.
Vitamin D	Beef, butter, eggs, milk, fish liver oils. Produced in the skin upon exposure to ultraviolet rays in sunlight. No plant source.	One of the most stable vitamins. Large doses may cause calcium deposits, poor bone growth in children, congenital defects.
Vitamin E	Widely distributed in foods. Abundant in vegetable oils and wheat germ.	Lost through oxidation during long cooking in open kettle. Overdose not known.
Vitamin K	Eggs, liver, cabbage, spinach, tomatoes. Produced by bacteria of intestine.	Destroyed by light and alkali. Absorption from intestine into blood depends upon normal fat absorption.
WATER-SOLUBLE VITAMINS		
Vitamin B_1 (Thiamine)	Meat, whole grains, liver, yeast, nuts, eggs, bran, soybeans, potatoes.	Not destroyed by cooking, but because it is water-soluble, may dissolve in cooking water. Not stored in body; daily supply needed.
Vitamin B_2 (Riboflavin)	Milk, cheese, liver, beef, eggs, fish.	Not destroyed by cooking acid foods. Unstable to light and alkali.
Niacin (Nicotinic acid)	Bran, eggs, yeast, liver and kidney, fish, whole wheat, potatoes, tomatoes. Can be synthesized from amino acid tryptophan.	Not destroyed by cooking, but may dissolve extensively in cooking water.
Vitamin B_6 (Pyridoxine)	Meat, liver, yeast, whole grains, fish, vegetables.	Stable except to light.
Vitamin B_{12} (Cyanocobalamin)	Meat, liver, eggs, milk, yeast.	Unstable to acid, alkali, light.
Vitamin C (Ascorbic acid)	Citrus fruits, tomatoes, potatoes, cabbage, green peppers, broccoli.	Least stable of the vitamins. Destroyed by heat, alkali, air. Dissolves in cooking water.

FUNCTION	DEFICIENCY SYMPTOMS	RECOMMENDED DAILY ALLOWANCE
Necessary for growth, tooth structure, night vision, healthy skin.	Slow growth, poor teeth and gums, night blindness, dry skin and eyes (lack of tears).	5000–8000 units for adult. 1500–5000 units for child.
Necessary for metabolism of calcium and phosphorous. Essential for normal bone and tooth development.	Rickets. Poor tooth and bone structure. Soft bones.	400 units.
Not definitely known for humans. Seems to help oxygen carriage in blood.	Not definitely known for humans.	Not established.
Necessary for blood clotting.	Slow blood clotting, anemia.	Not established. Often given to pregnant women and newborn infants since newborns lack bacteria which normally produce an adequate supply.
Necessary for carbohydrate metabolism, normal nerve function. Promotes growth.	Beriberi. Slow growth, poor nerve function, nervousness, fatigue, heart disease.	0.8 to 1.6 mg. for adult. 0.4 to 1.4 mg. for child.
Essential for metabolism in all cells.	Fatigue, sore skin and lips, bloodshot eyes, anemia.	1.2 to 2.0 mg. for adult. 0.6 to 2.0 mg. for child.
Necessary for growth, metabolism, normal skin.	Pellagra. Sore mouth, skin rash, indigestion, diarrhea, headache, mental disturbances.	13 to 20 mg. for adult. 6 to 22 mg. for child.
Functions in amino acid metabolism.	Dermatitis. Deficiency rare.	Not established.
Necessary for production of red blood cells and growth.	Pernicious anemia.	Not established.
Essential for cellular metabolism. Necessary for teeth, gums, bones, blood vessels, tissue repair.	Scurvy. Poor teeth, weak bones, sore and bleeding gums, easy bruising, poor wound healing.	70 to 100 mg. for adult. 30 to 80 mg. for child.

NOTE: Several other water-soluble vitamins are believed to be essential to human nutrition but are not so well understood as the above vitamins and their deficiency is less common.

Table 3.3 Minerals Most Often Deficient in Diets

MINERAL	RICH SOURCES	CHARACTERISTICS
Calcium	Dairy products, leafy vegetables.	Element most likely to be deficient in diet. Lack of vitamin D prevents use of calcium.
Phosphorus	Milk, liver, meat, beans, whole grains, cottage cheese, broccoli.	Most functions of any mineral in body. Diet adequate in calcium will usually contain sufficient phosphorous.
Iron	Liver, meat, shellfish, egg yolk, legumes, dried fruits.	Very little iron in milk; infant or child must have other source.
Iodine	Iodized salt.	Soil and water in some areas of U. S. very low in iodine. Only mineral in which deficiency in soil is reflected in dietary deficiency.
Fluorine	Drinking water in some areas of U. S.	Excess causes mottling of teeth.

active person might lose only 2.5 quarts of water through the four channels of water loss—kidneys, lungs, skin, and digestive tract. The same person might lose several times as much water if he were exercising vigorously on a hot day.

Thirst is usually an accurate indicator of water needs. However, a water intake slightly in excess of that dictated by thirst is advantageous for good kidney health.

DETERMINING DESIRABLE WEIGHT

Determining an individual's ideal weight is difficult, if not impossible. Body weight varies with sex, age, height, skeletal structure, rate of basal metabolism, and endocrine peculiarities. Since the so-called ideal, or average, individual does not exist, it is neither realistic nor possible to suggest an ideal weight applicable to all people. Consequently, in trying to arrive at a reasonable weight recommendation

FUNCTION	DEFICIENCY SYMPTOMS	RECOMMENDED DAILY ALLOWANCE
Building material for bones and teeth. Necessary for blood clotting and nerve function.	Rickets. Poor bone and tooth structure. Stunted growth. Cramps, twitching, and other symptoms of increased nerve irritability.	0.8–1.0 gm. for adult, 0.8–1.4 gm. for child, up to 2 gm. during pregnancy and nursing.
Essential in cell metabolism. Building material for bones and teeth. Serves as buffer to maintain proper pH of blood. Important in many enzyme systems including energy release.	Poorly developed teeth and bones, stunted growth, rickets, weakness, loss of weight.	1.5 gm. for adult, 1.0 gm. for child. Ratio of phosphorous to calcium should be 1.5:1 for adult and 1:1 for child.
Ingredients of hemoglobin, the oxygen-carrying pigment in red blood cells. Necessary for enzymes of cellular respiration.	Anemia (low oxygen-carrying capacity of blood).	10–15 mg. for adult, 8–15 mg. for child.
Basis of thyroid hormone.	Low metabolic rate. Goiter.	0.15–0.30 mg.
Strengthens bones and teeth.	Tooth decay.	1 part per million in drinking water.

for adults, the Food and Nutrition Board of the National Research Council has had to take a number of factors into consideration. Life insurance actuarial tables indicate that the most favorable health expectation is associated with the weight normally achieved at age twenty-two. Accordingly, it is recommended that the desirable weight for this age is the proper weight to maintain throughout adult life. In both sexes maximum body development is usually attained long before a person is twenty-two years old. Females attain such development when they are about eighteen years old and males when they are about twenty.

In Table 3.4 recommendations for weight are made on the bases of sex and height. Variations within each category are based on body build. In other words, a person with a smaller-than-average frame is expected to weigh somewhat less than the weight recommended for his given height, whereas an individual with a larger-than-average frame is expected to weigh more.

OVERWEIGHT AND OBESITY

Carrying extra pounds of either fat or muscle may adversely affect a person's total fitness, his personal life, and his social and economic position. Extra pounds of fat are more damaging than extra pounds of muscle because muscle supports itself. It is better, however, not to carry extra weight of either kind.

A distinction should be made between the words *obesity* and *overweight*. Obesity is "an excessive deposition of fat beyond what is considered normal for a given age, sex, and body build." Weight, on the other hand, is "a quantity of heaviness." A person who is overweight, then, is not necessarily overly fat; he is merely overly heavy. A person who is overweight may also be defined as any person weighing more than is recommended in Table 3.4.

Overweight

Body weight includes fat, muscle, and bone. If any of these is greater than normal, a person may be overweight. He may not be obese but he may have excessively large bone structure or heavy muscular development. It is also possible for an individual of average weight to be excessively fat if his muscular and bone structures are relatively small.

There is no easy way of accurately measuring a person's body fat in relation to his total weight. Generally, however, if a person is 20 percent above the desirable weight given in Table 3.4, he can be rather sure he is obese. Another simple indicator of fatness is the ruler test. When one is lying flat on his back and is relaxed, the surface of the abdomen between the flare of the ribs and the pubis (the bone directly below the navel when standing) is normally flat or slightly concave. A ruler placed on the abdomen parallel to the vertical axis should touch both ribs and pubis.

Table 3.4 Desirable Weights

HEIGHT IN INCHES[a]	WEIGHT IN POUNDS		
	MEN	WOMEN	
60		109 ±	9[b]
62		115 ±	9
64	133 ± 11	122 ±	10
66	142 ± 12	129 ±	10
68	151 ± 14	136 ±	10
70	159 ± 14	144 ±	11
72	167 ± 15	152 ±	12
74	175 ± 15		

[a]Heights and weights are without shoes and other clothing.
[b]Desirable weight for a small-framed woman of this height would be approximately 109 lb. minus 9 lb., or a total of 100 lb.; for a average-framed woman, 109 lb.; for a large-framed woman, 118 lb.
SOURCE: Food and Nutrition Board, National Research Council.

Obesity

If someone wants to lose a substantial amͦ
he must limit his food intake. For an obese person exercise aͪ
activity are not substitutes for limitations on eating. Because oͭ
plications which might arise in body systems such as the heart anͩ
circulatory system, obese individuals should start on programs combin-
ing exercise and reductions in food intake only in consultation with a
physician.

Inactivity is, however, a major cause of obesity. If one rides
in a car, instead of walks, to school or work each day and if the distance covered is about two and one-half miles, he may gain a pound
of body fat in about thirteen days. In most cases excess weight can be
reduced if one exercises without increasing food intake. Strenuous,
programmed, consistent exercise leads to increases in food intake, but
these increases remain within the range of what is being used by the
body. The weight of stored fat is reduced, used, and displaced by increased muscle activity. Many individuals do not overeat, they underexercise. Remember, walking two and a half miles to school or work
each day can use up a pound in about thirteen days.

In general, obesity results either from faulty metabolism or
from faulty regulation of the diet or appetite. Fat cells in adipose tissue (the fat deposit of the body) are in a continual state of flux. Within
these cells, fats are continually being built up for storage and broken
down for metabolism. Each individual has a unique metabolic rate.
Some use this stored food faster or slower than others do and, accordingly, have a higher or lower rate of metabolism. Differences in
rate are the result of specific hormone and enzyme activities in the
body. Metabolic rate is influenced by inherited or developmental differences and can be altered by disease in the pituitary or thyroid
glands. A faulty metabolism may cause either overweight or under-
weight.

Generally, obesity is caused by a person's failure to regulate
his food intake. Appetite control is very important to the ability to
control weight. Appetite is controlled by a small area in the brain
called the "appetite center," or "appestat." The center consists of two
parts, two small groups of brain cells called *nuclei* (Figure 3.1). When
one set of cells is stimulated, a person wants to eat; when the other
set is stimulated, he feels satisfied. Thus the appestat controls the appetite in a manner similar to that of a thermostat in controlling the
temperature of a room.

Scientists do not know how the two centers of the appestat
become activated. They may be activated by the glucose level (blood
sugar level) in the blood, by changes in body temperature, or by the
level of amino acids in the blood.

Scientists do know, however, that there are nerve connections
between the appetite center and the cortex of the brain. Thus appetite

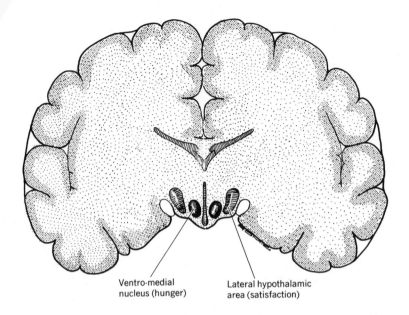

Ventro-medial
nucleus (hunger)

Lateral hypothalamic
area (satisfaction)

Figure 3.1 Hypothalamic nuclei regulating appetite and satiety.

may be controlled not only by body functions but may also be controlled consciously by the brain. Perhaps it is possible for people to "learn" how much food they like before they are satisfied. Appetite, then, may be controlled by learned behavior and emotional factors, as well as by chemical factors.

Emotional factors which may affect appetite include worry, tension, frustration, and conflicts in interpersonal relations. For some people, eating seems to compensate for domestic troubles, financial problems, illness in the family, social upsets, and anxiety over schoolwork or a pending business deal. For others, eating is a pleasant break from a monotonous routine.

Research has shown, too, that inheritance plays a part in the "setting" of a person's appestat. One person may have a "higher setting" than another person and require more food to feel satisfied.

There are other factors which do not directly affect appetite but which may lead to obesity. These include a person's economic status, his occupation, the state of his health, and his age. People with limited amounts of money, for example, often buy inexpensive foods. Such foods are usually high in carbohydrates, sugars and starches. People whose jobs involve the preparation and serving of food sometimes become habitual samplers and nibblers. This is true of people who work in candy shops, restaurants, and bakeries. It may also be true of housewives, who spend much of their time buying and preparing food.

When people fall victim to disease or become disabled, their ability to engage in physical activity may become severely impaired. In that case they must change their eating habits or gain weight. Age also affects weight. Sixty percent of American men in their fifties are obese. As a person grows older, his basal metabolic rate drops and the level of his physical activity diminishes. However, he may eat as much as he did when he was younger. If long-established eating patterns are not changed, obesity results.

Regardless of the underlying causes of obesity, the basic problem confronting an obese person is simply one of taking in more calories than are needed for all his activities—basic metabolism, heat loss, work, and exercise. Unused calories from any source are stored in the body as fat. Each pound of stored fat represents about 3500 calories. Calories are either used or stored. Obesity increases in relation to the amount of stored calories.

Effects of Obesity

Life insurance records show that obese individuals are poorer risks than people of normal weight. Their life expectancy is shorter; in fact, a person's chances of dying at an early age increase in direct proportion to the amount of excess weight he carries. So do his chances of having certain diseases.

Respiratory difficulties are common in people who are obese. The more weight a person has in his chest wall, the more work he must expend to breathe. Obese people show a higher frequency of respiratory infections than people of normal weight. They are also more likely to build up carbon dioxide in their blood since it is much harder to breathe correctly when obese.

Blood pressure generally rises with weight increase (and often returns to normal with comparable weight loss). An obese person with high blood pressure (hypertension) runs a greater risk of coronary heart disease than does a nonobese person with hypertension. For every pound of added fat tissue, there is an additional three-fourths of a mile of blood vessels; this adds to the stress on the heart.

Obesity is dangerous for other reasons, too. It complicates pregnancy; toxemia and stillbirths are more prevalent among obese people than they are among people of normal weight. Gall bladder diseases, diabetes, digestive diseases, and nephritis are also more prevalent. Obesity can aggravate conditions such as varicose veins, osteoarthritis and other bone and joint diseases, congestive heart failure, and angina pectoris. Fat accumulating around internal vital organs tends to crowd them. Obese people run an increased risk when they have surgery.

Obese people frequently complain of "that tired feeling," because they must exert effort to carry unnecessary body fat. Obese people are also less agile, have more balancing problems, and move more slowly than do people of normal weight, and they have less tolerance for exercise. They tend to have more accidents, too.

Of course, excess weight is unattractive. Fat people of both sexes frequently show "stretch marks" on the skin, which may not disappear with weight loss.

Exercise and Weight Control

Weight reduction is the outcome of a negative calorie balance. In other words, to lose weight, a person must consume fewer calories than he uses. In any weight control program, caloric intake must be judged in relation to energy needs.

Physical activity is necessary for weight loss. However, as pointed out by Mayer,[1] it is not necessary or even desirable to attempt to reduce 1 pound of body weight in one exercise or sport session: this represents a large expenditure of energy. "A half hour of handball or squash a day would be equivalent to 19 pounds of body weight per year."

Appetite usually increases in proportion to increase in activity. However, inactive individuals who engage in slight activity experience an exaggerated increase in appetite and, thus, gain weight. Physical inactivity is an underlying characteristic of obese individuals. Young people who are obese are inactive youths. Often, they overeat because they underexercise. The intensity of physical activity is one of the most important factors influencing weight control. Every year, many Americans find out that it is impossible to reduce weight or to "diet" without increasing physical activity. Consequently, people who want to maintain a desirable weight or who are trying to reduce their weight to a desirable level must plan physical activities in which to engage regularly throughout the week.

As pointed out previously, an increase in metabolic rate is incurred during physical activity and is the main cause of energy loss, or calorie use. However, in a physically active individual the increased metabolic rate persists for several hours after completion of physical activity, even though the individual is resting. Exercise physiologists have shown that a higher metabolic rate in an active individual may persist for as long as six hours after completion of a period of active physical activity. An individual who exercises daily can lose four to five pounds a year from the increase in metabolic rate alone; this does not take into consideration the energy cost of the activity itself.

[1]Jean Mayer, "Exercise and Weight Control," *Exercise and Fitness* (A collection of Papers Presented at the Colloquium on Exercise and Fitness), University of Illinois, Urbana, Illinois, 1960, Chapter 12, pp. 110–121.

SUMMARY

I. The human body is a very efficient energy-conve.

   A. Energy, or the capacity to do work, exists in tw

     1. Potential energy—latent energy, or chemical e

     2. Kinetic energy—active forms of energy doing v

   B. The unit for expressing the energy content of foot calorie, or kilocalorie.

II. Energy Requirements and Food

   A. All the chemical reactions which require energy make up the metabolism of the body.

   B. An individual's energy expenditure is his basal metabolic rate (BMR).

   C. In addition to the energy needed for basal metabolism, a widely varying quantity of energy is needed for everyday activities.

III. Foods

   A. Foods fulfill several of the body's important requirements:

     1. They are sources of energy.

     2. They supply materials for growth and replacement of worn or damaged cells.

     3. They are needed for manufacture of cellular products such as enzymes and hormones.

   B. Foods may be classified into three categories:

     1. Carbohydrates

       a. Sugars (monosaccharides and dissaccharides).

       b. Starches (polysaccharides).

       c. Carbohydrates are the most important sources of energy available to the body.

     2. Fats

       a. Have the highest energy content of any known food.

       b. Serve as body's reservoir for long-term storage of energy.

       c. Are important to the membranes of all cells.

       d. Apparently, humans must have small quantities of fats in their diets if the fat-soluble vitamins are to be absorbed into the blood.

     3. Proteins

       a. Of the three groups of foods (carbohydrates, fats, and proteins), the proteins are the most essential to life.

       b. Proteins consist of chains of amino acids. There are twenty common amino acids; eight of these are essential to human life. If the remaining twelve amino acids are not obtained through the diet, they can be produced within the body.

       c. Proteins containing the eight essential amino acids in significant quantities are said to be of high biological value.

    d. Proteins are of primary importance to normal growth and maintenance of the human body.

IV. Essential Substances Found in Foods

  A. Vitamins

    1. Vitamins are essential to the execution of specific chemical reactions.

    2. Vitamins are not sources of energy.

    3. Some people now believe that as many as thirteen minerals are necessary for optimum human health.

  B. Water

    1. No other chemical compound serves the body in so many distinct and vital functions as does water.

    2. Water is the medium in which all chemical reactions of metabolism take place.

    3. A person's daily requirement depends greatly on the temperature of his environment (room temperature) and on the amount of physical activity he engages in.

    4. Water intake should be slightly in excess of thirst for good kidney health.

V. Determining Desirable Weight

  A. Determining the ideal weight for an individual is difficult, if not impossible. Body weight varies with sex, age, height, skeletal structure, rate of basal metabolism, and endocrine peculiarities.

  B. Life insurance tables indicate that the most favorable health expectation is the weight normally achieved at age twenty-two.

VI. Overweight and Obesity

  A. Obesity—an excessive deposition of fat beyond what is considered normal for a given age, sex, and body build.

  B. Overweight—an overweight person is overly heavy but not necessarily overly fat; he may have excessively large bone structure or heavy muscular development.

  C. Obesity may be caused by faulty metabolism.

  D. Obesity is usually caused by a person's failure to regulate his food intake.

    1. Appetite Control

      a. Appetite is controlled by the "appetite center," or "appestat," in the brain.

      b. Appetite may be controlled consciously by the brain. People may "learn" how much to eat. Thus, learned behavior and emotional factors may affect appetite.

      c. Appetite and the "appestat" may be affected by inheritance.

2. Factors which do not directly affect appetite but which may lead to obesity:
   a. Economic status.
   b. Occupation.
   c. State of health.
   d. Age.
E. Regardless of the underlying causes of obesity, the basic problem confronting an obese person is simply one of taking in more calories than are needed for all his activities.
F. Effects of Obesity
   1. The prevalence of certain diseases and the danger of dying at an early age increase in direct proportion to the amount of excess weight.
      a. Respiratory difficulties are common.
      b. Blood pressure usually rises with weight increase; this increases the risk of coronary heart disease.
      c. Obesity complicates pregnancy (toxemia and stillbirths are prevalent).
      d. Obesity can aggravate existing conditions.
      e. Obese people run an increased risk when they have surgery.
      f. Fat accumulates around internal organs and crowds them.
   2. Obesity leads to tiredness because people must exert effort to carry unnecessary body fat.
   3. Obese individuals are less agile, have more balancing problems, and tend to have more accidents than people of normal weight.
   4. Excess weight is unattractive.
VII. Exercise and Weight Control
   A. Weight reduction is the outcome of a negative calorie balance.
   B. Physical activity is necessary for weight loss.
   C. People who want to maintain a desirable weight or who are trying to reduce their weight to a desirable level must plan physical activities in which to engage regularly throughout the week.

QUESTIONS FOR REVIEW

1. Distinguish between Recommended Daily Allowances and Minimum Daily Requirements. Do these vary among people?
2. Using the reference charts, calculate your own desirable weight for your age and height; then calculate your caloric needs for maintaining this weight.

3. How does one go about adjusting his caloric intake to match his physical activity? Why should this be done?
4. How might regular eating habits become a significant problem for an older person? What steps can be taken to avoid this problem?
5. Define overweight. Contrast overweight with obesity. What are the differences in the meanings of the two words?
6. Explain the ruler test. Perform this test on yourself. What are the results?
7. What factors control appetite?

Chapter 4

VALUES OF TOTAL FITNESS

The means of achieving total fitness must be planned and evaluated in terms of needs. The goals of total fitness programs should include the improvement of a person's vigor, endurance, body build, and his increased participation in his social groups and his society in general.

Total fitness is valuable for both males and females. Thus all of the discussions in this book are directed toward both sexes. Contrary to some common thought, women who participate in exercise programs and sports do not develop large muscles. Programs which overdevelop specific muscles are unhealthy for both men and women.

Exercise improves the figure by "normalizing" it, or causing it to become better proportioned. If the arms or legs are too heavy, exercise slims them; if they are too thin, exercise develops them. Even American female Olympic athletes, such as skiers, track participants, gymnasts, and skaters have feminine body builds.

Although women are usually neither as strong nor as powerful as men, they have better flexibility, poise, and grace. They enjoy participating in sports aimed at developing a beautiful, womanly figure— one that is slender, graceful, and has curves in the right places. Most beautiful women participate in daily exercise programs and in sports.

PHYSICAL GROWTH AND DEVELOPMENT

Muscular activity stimulates the growth and development of the body. Growth is defined as observable increases in general body size, including changes in height and weight, and alterations in tissue makeup and in the internal organs. The importance of physical activity for the proper growth and development of children is virtually unquestioned.

The study of growth is complicated by the close relationships among heredity, nutrition, and muscular activity in affecting the formation of the body. The *configuration* (general form) of the body is determined largely by heredity. Muscular activity, however, is valuable because it provides the means through which the body can develop to its optimum inherited potential.

A well-developed body is necessary for many reasons. Fully developed bones and muscles provide protection against injury. They enable a person to perform the necessary activities of daily life, and they increase his endurance both for work and for recreational activities. Furthermore, in our culture a well-formed, or well-developed, body is appreciated for aesthetic reasons.

A significant study done by Buskirk[1] shows the effect of athletic activity on development. In the study X rays of the forearms and hands of a group of nationally ranked tennis players were compared with X rays of a group of non-tennis-playing soldiers. The X rays of the tennis players revealed increases in breadth in the distal end of the ulna. They also revealed a much greater development of other bones and muscles in the dominant arm (arm in which the racket is held) than in the nondominant arm. The differences between the dominant and nondominant arms of tennis players who have achieved an exceptional level of performance indicates that long-term muscular activity affects structural development.

AGING PROCESSES

A person's health is determined by the vitality and health of the cells in his body. One of the factors which determines cell health

[1]Elsworth R. Buskirk, Lange, K. Anderson, and Joseph Brozek, "Unilateral Activity and Bone and Muscle Development in the Forearm," *Research Quarterly*, Vol. 27, No. 2 (May, 1965), pp. 127–131.

is total fitness. A person's body ages as the vitality of his cells declines. Under optimum conditions of energy supply, oxygen supply, waste removal, and periods of functioning and rest, the cells—and, thus, the body—tend to live longer. Therefore, two people of the same chronological age may be of different *biological ages* if one person is more fit than the other. By studying large groups of individuals, scientists have been able to estimate someone's biological age, without considering his chronological age.

Biological age is measured by changes in the structure and functioning of the major body systems. Within these systems, different physiological functions change at different rates. Some changes take place rapidly, but others appear to be age-resistant. The biological-aging process can be accelerated by a deficient food supply, inactivity, disuse or loss of function of organs, and external factors such as infection, traumatic injury, and physical irritation. These factors can lead to deterioration of the body, disease, and *premature death* (death prior to estimations for the general population).

Man's struggle for a better life has brought about impressive improvements in his living conditions: cleaner homes and working places, regulation of working hours, the opportunities for recuperative rest and sleep, and striking advances in nutrition. Such improvements have caused tremendous changes in man's physical condition. Medical science has relieved humans of epidemic diseases such as cholera, plague, smallpox, typhus, and diphtheria. Recently it has almost conquered tuberculosis. The elimination of these diseases along with a lowered infant mortality rate have increased the average American's life span. In the last one hundred years, for example, the life expectancy of American males has been extended from forty to over sixty-seven years and that of American females from forty to over seventy-four years.

Because life expectancy has increased, people now die of diseases which used to be uncommon. Today, deaths are frequently caused by *degenerative conditions*, diseases which cause changes in the structure and functioning of the body: arteriosclerosis (hardening of the arteries), coronary thrombosis (cardiac infarction), cerebral thrombosis (stroke), and cancer of various organs. These diseases usually become manifest only after the continuous, prolonged action of various harmful factors. Therefore, they occur more frequently than they did in the past because many people live long enough to fall victim to them.

Exercise physiologists have shown that physical exercise, if it is sufficiently intensive, can greatly delay the various phenomena of aging. It can help a person avoid decrease in muscle mass, diminished oxygen intake, reduced heat production, and fall in total blood quantity. All are exaggerated by lack of sufficient physical activity.

Physical exercises also increase overall cerebral activities.

They stimulate the neural controls of metabolism, respiration, blood circulation, and digestion. They also stimulate the activities of the glands of internal secretion. A combination of alert mental activity and physical exercise is the best method of preserving, for as long as possible, the ability of the brain cells to act at a high level.

The control of the phenomena of aging—the fight for longevity —should begin as early as possible, before the body becomes completely developed. Premature biological aging is difficult to control once it has set in. That is why the habits of physical exercise and total fitness should be developed in early childhood.

An example of someone who has retained youthfulness is the woman of fifty who looks and acts like a woman of thirty. If she prolongs her good looks and vitality by exercising regularly, a middle-aged woman may find that her older years are her happiest ones.

DEGENERATIVE BODY CONDITIONS

The first signs of degenerative body conditions usually appear as premature damage to the cardiovascular and respiratory systems. Such damage is caused by poor diet, smoking, heredity, congenital defects, and lack of physical activity. Socioeconomic pressures, emotional tensions, anxieties, and frustrations are contributing factors.

The Respiratory System and Breathing

The respiratory system (Figure 4.1) contains the organs in which oxygen and carbon dioxide are exchanged. In the lungs air breathed in is processed; also, oxygen is removed and transferred to the blood stream for distribution throughout the body. Figure 4.2 illustrates the distribution process: Air comes into the lungs; the oxygen is removed from the air by diffusion, fed into the *hemoglobin* in the red blood cells, and sent through the bloodstream for distribution. When the red blood cells reach the capillaries, the oxygen diffuses out to the tissues. The carbon dioxide is picked up and carried back to the lungs where it diffuses into the air and is carried out of the body.

The atmospheric air breathed in by humans is approximately 21 percent oxygen; the percentage rarely varies. What does vary is the amount of air a person is able to process through his lungs. If the lungs can't process an adequate supply of air, they do not extract enough oxygen to produce energy.

Expansion and contraction of the lungs are completely dependent on the muscles of the rib cage and diaphragm. If a person is exercising, the muscles of the rib cage contract when he inhales. This contraction expands the rib cage and creates a large capacity for air in the lung cavity (almost a vacuum). The outside air, pushed by atmospheric

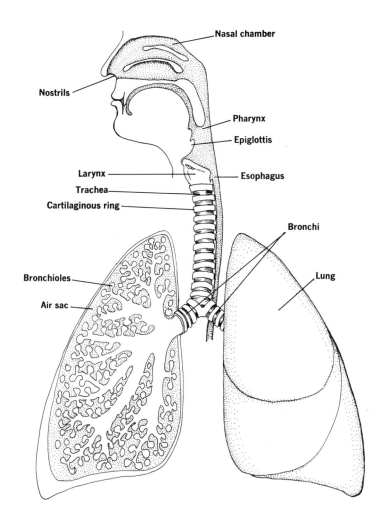

Figure 4.1 The respiratory system.

pressure, rushes in. When the person exhales, the muscles of the rib cage, aided by the natural elasticity of the lungs and chest wall, recoil and actually force the air out against atmospheric pressure. Thus inhaling causes air to be pushed into the lungs by atmospheric pressure; exhaling causes it to be pushed out by the muscles.

When he rests, a person breathes at a minimal rate and the rhythmical movement of air is controlled by contraction (inhalation) and relaxation (exhalation) of the diaphragm. The normal respiration rate at rest ranges from fourteen to twenty breaths per minute; the average is seventeen. At rest all persons consume about the same amount

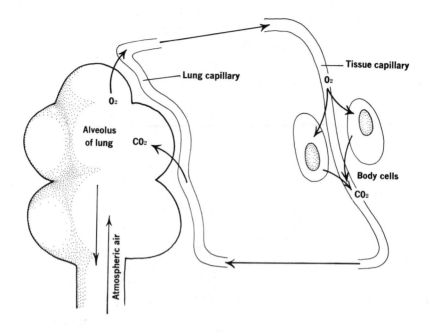

Figure 4.2 Diagram illustrating the exchange of gases between the lungs and the body cells.

of oxygen. Consequently, everyone inhales and exhales about the same amount of air; the amount contains more than enough oxygen.

When a person becomes physically active, the amount of air he can inhale and exhale is limited by two factors. First, the muscles of the rib cage must create a large vacuum into which the lungs may expand. Second, the muscles must recoil and squeeze back into a small area. When people exercise, they condition the muscles of the rib cage and diaphragm and, thus, increase their capability for inhaling and exhaling air. When more air can be inhaled, there is more oxygen; when more air can be exhaled, there is less carbon dioxide.

The amount of air which a person can process in a specific amount of time is a significant indicator of his physical condition. Any deterioration of the lung tissues reduces the lung's capacity to process air. During the aging process, the normal decrease in the gas-exchange capabilities of a person's lungs is largely responsible for his decreasing physical ability. Adequate physical activity can delay this biological-aging process. Active lungs retain their abilities for many more years than do relatively inactive lungs. Insufficient activity, air pollution, irritations, and disease organisms may cause premature damage which decreases the effectiveness of the lungs to the point where specific symptoms of certain diseases appear.

EMPHYSEMA

It is sometimes difficult to explain and discuss specific lung diseases because one lung disease coexists with or leads to another disease. Even physicians may have difficulty differentiating among the diseases. In general, however, the most common diseases associated with deterioration of the lung tissues are *emphysema* and the condition which often leads to it, *bronchitis.*

Emphysema is a degenerative condition in which the lung tissues lose their elasticity and the walls of the air sacs (Figure 4.1) break down. Emphysema restricts the transfer of gases (oxygen and carbon dioxide) to and from the blood. The lungs of people suffering from emphysema are stretched, broken, and swollen. They have usually been destroyed by coughing caused by smoking, asthma, bronchitis, or even tuberculosis. Such destruction takes place readily if the lungs have not been kept active through physical exercise.

The stretching of the lungs causes them to lose their elasticity. Thus air begins to accumulate in them, especially in areas well supported by the muscles of the rib cage. As the air accumulates, the ability of the lungs to push it out is reduced. The lungs become less and less active. Emphysema finally results in death.

BRONCHITIS

Chronic bronchitis is an inflamation of the lining of the bronchial tubes (Figure 4.1). When the bronchi become inflamed, they are easily infected. Inflamed and infected bronchi impede air flow to and from the lungs, causing labored breathing and heavy mucus, or phlegm, to be coughed up. A brief attack of acute bronchitis with fever, coughing, and spitting occurs with severe colds. In *chronic bronchitis* coughing and spitting continue for months and return periodically.

The Cardiovascular System and Circulation

From the lungs, oxygen goes directly into the bloodstream. The lungs contain millions of small air sacs (Figure 4.1), called *alveoli,* around which the blood flows. The oxygen moves by *diffusion* from an area of high pressure in the alveoli to an area of lower pressure in the red blood cells.

The factors in the blood which affect health include the number of red blood cells (normally about 4.5 to 5.5 million per cubic millimeter of blood) and the amount of hemoglobin in these cells. Even if the lungs can process large amounts of oxygen, the body tissues can receive only limited amounts if the red cells or hemoglobin which deliver the oxygen are in short supply. A totally fit individual has more blood than one who is not fit. Because he has more hemoglobin and more blood plasma (the fluid portion of the blood), which contain the red blood cells, his total volume of blood is greater. Tests show that men in good physical condition invariably have a larger blood supply than average men of comparable size.

The heart takes the oxygen-filled blood from the lungs and pumps it throughout the body. It also takes carbon-dioxide-filled blood from the body and pumps it into the lungs. The heart works harder, faster, and less efficiently in a nonexerciser than in a totally fit individual. Someone who is in condition and is active on a regular basis may have a resting heart rate of between 55 and 60 beats per minute. An inactive nonexerciser may have a resting heart rate of 70 or more. If the heart rate of a fit individual is 60 beats per minute, his heart beats 3,600 beats per hour, or 86,400 beats per 24 hours. If the heart rate of a nonexerciser is 80 beats per minute, his heart rate is 4,800 beats per hour, or 115,200 beats per day. The nonexerciser, then, forces his heart to beat nearly 30,000 more times each day.

The heart of a totally fit person can beat less because the decreased heart rate is more than compensated for by increased blood volume. In other words, each pump of the heart moves a greater volume of blood. Also, as the volume of blood increases, the body builds more blood vessels, especially in the muscles. Called *increased tissue vascularization,* this is a remarkable phenomenon which delays aging by keeping tissues alive and healthy.

In the totally fit individual, blood pressure is usually lower than in the nonexerciser, because blood vessels are more pliable and have less resistance to blood flow. Exercise improves existing blood vessels and, thus, reduces blood pressure. However, a person retains reduced blood pressure only as long as he remains in condition. Reduced heart rate, vascularization, and reduced blood pressure are essential in building endurance and in combating fatigue. They contribute to an increased blood supply which saturates tissues, such as cardiac muscles, with oxygen and carries away more wastes. Oxygen saturation is extremely vital to the health of the heart, the most important muscle in the body.

Regular exercise can help prevent heart disease. It is uncommon for an athlete who has maintained a vigorous exercise program throughout life to develop coronary heart disease. Furthermore, studies of former athletes who have had coronary heart disease (any destructive process involving blood vessels conducting blood to the heart muscle) show that these athletes engaged in less vigorous exercise than did other athletes. If a person does have a heart attack, his chances of survival are greatly increased if his blood vessels are healthy enough to supply the heart tissue with large amounts of energy-producing oxygen.

The National Heart Institute and the American Heart Association agree that one of the major causes of *atherosclerosis,* (a decrease of inside diameter of blood vessels because inner walls become thickened by deposits of fat), a major cardiovascular disease, is lack of exercise. Many studies indicate that the chemical cholesterol is greatly responsible for atherosclerosis. Exercise helps the body to maintain normal levels of cholesterol despite relatively high intakes of fat. Vigorous physical activity three days per week for five weeks produces significant decreases in plasma cholesterol. Such decreases are linked to the reduced blood pressure attained through exercise. High blood pressure stimulates the production of cholesterol in the liver. This, in turn, increases cholesterol levels in the blood which accelerate the formation of cholesterol plagues and lead to atherosclerosis.

There are many factors (diet, heredity, smoking, obesity, lack of physical activity) linked to the enormously widespread incidence of degenerative cardiovascular conditions. It is difficult to single out any one factor and say that it is the major cause of such conditions. However, the individual who seems to have a good chance of suffering a heart attack is one who eats too much, smokes too much, worries too much, and gets insufficient exercise. Such a person, especially if he comes from a family with a history of heart conditions, is "a heart attack waiting for a place to happen."

Physicians, physiologists, and, recently, the general public have begun to accept the idea that lifetime muscular activity will lead to a decrease in the incidence of degenerative cardiovascular conditions. Dr. Paul Dudley White, the well-known cardiologist who has long been an advocate of exercise, said recently, "I believe that the physiological effect of regular exercise throughout one's life will probably, in time, be proved one of the best antidotes against the alarming development of the epidemic of coronary thrombosis and high blood pressure in this country." He added, "One of the faults of our current civilization is that our young adults at about the age of twenty-five become 'too busy' to exercise. Yet, for the next two decades of their lives, they probably need it even more than when they were children."

TOTAL FITNESS AND MUSCULAR ACTIVITY

As you have learned, there are three kinds of muscles in the body: *skeletal*, which provide the force for the movement of bones (these muscles are discussed more fully in Chapter 2); *smooth*, which provide lining for blood vessels and are found in the walls of the digestive tract; and *cardiac*, which are found only in the heart.

Exercise and the Skeletal Muscles

The skeletal muscles (muscles of the arms, legs, back, etc.) produce movement by contracting to become shorter and thicker and by relaxing to elongate back to their original length. Nearly all of the skeletal muscles work in pairs. Results of this paired cooperation include movements such as walking, running, and climbing.

Many exercises and physical activities affect the skeletal muscles. Some are aimed solely at building, or enlarging, the muscles, but others are aimed at total fitness.

Sports which contribute to total fitness include bicycling, running, jogging, swimming, and tennis. Such sports cause the muscles to grow longer and leaner so more of the cells are closer to the blood vessels. They also help to create new blood vessels. People in good condition have bodies in which almost all the parts are well supplied with blood vessels. Of course, an individual must possess sufficient muscular strength to support his own body weight easily before he uses his muscles for any other physical activity. The bulding of muscles up to the point where a person can perform in a total fitness program is the value of muscle-strengthening exercises.

Exercise and the Smooth Muscles

The smooth muscles are less affected by physical activity than are the skeletal and cardiac muscles. As you have seen, however, the elasticity of the muscles and their ability to contract are greatly increased by physical activity. Exercise also improves the performance of the smooth muscles. For example, it helps the muscles of the digestive tract to increase the efficiency of digestive processes, to move waste materials along, and to aid in the activity of the bowel.

At one time people believed that any muscular activity engaged in directly after eating had a detrimental effect on digestion. This has been found to be untrue. Moderate exercise undertaken directly after a meal does not interfere with the digestive processes. A person who engages in vigorous muscular activity immediately after a meal may, however, find that his ability to perform is impaired. For this reason people should limit, but not avoid, muscular activities immediately after eating.

BODY FLEXIBILITY

Flexibility—the ability to move freely in various directions—involves a wide range of body motions. Today, people spend almost 95 percent of their time sitting. This causes the muscles of the shoulders, chest, back, and legs to shorten and tighten. Shortening and weakening of the body muscles are the major causes of low back pains. In a recent medical report involving 5,000 individuals who had low back pain, 80 percent were unable to pass some of the simplest tests for muscular strength.

Good body flexibility permits greater freedom of body movements and helps prevent muscle injuries such as torn ligaments, sprains, and muscle separations. A total fitness program improves flexibility because muscles, ligaments, and connecting tissues are repeatedly stretched.

BODY COORDINATION

A coordinated person is able to use the proper muscles with the proper force at the proper time. No one is quite sure how to transform clumsy body movements into smooth and skillful ones. Research indicates that coordination involves specific muscles. Often, the learning of the skills and abilities needed to perform one task cannot be transferred to another task. Furthermore, coordination develops only with repeated practice.

The most significant point in coordination development is that muscular activity increases an individual's ability to perform more muscular activity. The only way to improve a specific physical skill is to impose specific demands on the muscles involved in the skill. After a person learns to perform a skill by practicing it, he does not lose the skill; he can perform it when necessary. However, a person's level of coordination and ability in performing the skill always depend on continuing training and practice.

MENTAL VALUES OF TOTAL FITNESS

The central nervous system consists of the spinal cord and the brain, which is made up of the *cerebellum*, the *cerebrum*, and the *brain stem* (Figure 4.3). The spinal cord and primitive portions of the brain, the brain stem and cerebellum, are shared by all higher animals, such as pigeons, dogs, and man. The cerebrum (Figure 4.4) controls mental activities which belong only to the human brain. Because of the cerebrum, humans have the ability to remember, to form judgments, to form symbols, words, languages, and ideas, to reason, and to control their skeletal muscles. Predictably, destruction of portions of the cerebrum results in losses of these mental functions.

Every use of the body involves related portions of the nervous system. Voluntary movements, especially the learning of skills, are functions of the cerebrum. With or without interference or direction from this "thinking" cerebrum, repeated use of the centers of the nervous system improves the effectiveness with which they mobilize the inner organs and systems to support better functioning of the whole body.

Approximately 40 percent of the nerve fibers connecting a nerve to a muscle are actually *sensory fibers* which carry nerve impulses from muscles, tendons, and their related joints into the spinal cord and on to the brain. Called *proprioception*, or *kinethesia*, this "muscle sense" provides the mind with its understanding of stretch, tension,

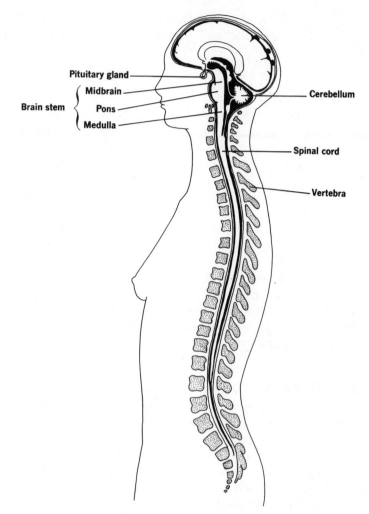

Figure 4.3 Central nervous system.

movement, body position, and the third dimension. Judged only by the eyes, a sphere seems to be merely a circle. After the hands have closed around it, however, the concept of roundness becomes apparent. The concept of a spherical sun would be inconceivable to a person whose hands had never clutched a ball. Without the proprioceptive sensations which arise from activity in muscles and joints, our "abstract, inner world" of concepts would be flat and unreal.

Physical activity is important to the human mind because every movement, every body position, and every tension in a muscle, tendon, and joint help to contribute to the formation of concepts and ideas. The high degree of common sense exhibited by many relatively uneducated people who work with their hands may exist because such

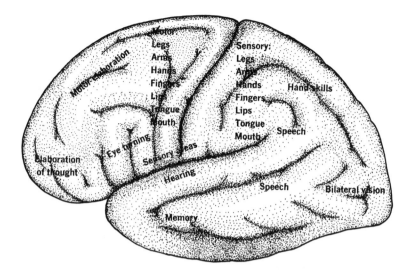

Figure 4.4 Cerebral function map.

people are richly supplied with "muscle sense." Perhaps the unexpected lack of common sense sometimes displayed by people who have been educated through books is caused by a lack of "muscle sense." Today, more and more people work in occupations which involve thought and abstraction. For modern people, then, participation in sports and other physical activities may offer one of the few available "retreats into reality."

The degree of success a person attains depends on the quality of his performance. Sports and other physical activities represent "life speeded up." For example, in tennis the body must move faster and the mind make decisions more rapidly than in ordinary life. Thus in physical competition hundreds of decisions are made and executed in the amount of time allowed for ten decisions in ordinary life. Even more important, such decisions must be made in the heat of emotion brought on by the competition, and they should be made fairly and efficiently. In this sense competition is an important stimulus to the body; the muscles must perform efficiently, and the mind must make quick, accurate decisions while maintaining control over the emotions.

RESISTANCE TO COMMUNICABLE DISEASES

Hypothetically, a person in perfect health would be immune to all communicable diseases and would be able to resist the degenerative changes which come with age. Since the relationship between total fitness and physical degeneration has already been discussed, we shall now discuss only the relationship between fitness and communicable diseases (diseases which are passed from person to person).

Advocates of physical fitness have long felt that physical training and conditioning provide a degree of resistance to communicable diseases. Physical training per se does not increase the body's resistance to specific diseases. Resistance is increased, however, by general factors related to fitness: good nutrition, the body's ability to ward off fatigue, and its ability to maintain an effective control over blood pressure and the circulatory system in general.

Physical exercise increases body resistance to oxygen debt, overheating, and chilling and, thus, helps the body to resist disease processes. There is also increased resistance to some poisons, such as trichlorethylamine, but not to others, such as strychnine, carbon monoxide, and potassium cyanide. In regard to infection, experiments show that processes important to the control of disease are more active in the trained individual than they are in the untrained individual.

If physical exercise is to help the body resist disease, it must be of optimum intensity and duration. Too little or too much physical activity fails not only to produce the desired resistance but it might, in some cases, result in decreased resistance.

In discussions about the effects of physical activity, the body is usually divided into areas and systems. However, most physical activity improves and promotes the efficiency of the whole organism and is essential for the proper functioning and maintenance of all systems of the body. A balanced program of total fitness is of profound importance to the life of any individual.

SUMMARY

    I. The means of achieving total fitness must be planned and evaluated in terms of individual needs.

   II. Physical Growth and Development

      A. Growth refers to observable increases in general body size.

         1. Changes in height and weight.

         2. Alterations in the tissue makeup.

         3. Changes in the internal organs.

      B. Muscular activity stimulates growth and development of the body.

      C. A well-developed body is considered necessary for many reasons:

         1. Protection against injury.

         2. Performance of daily activities.

         3. Endurance.

         4. Aesthetic reasons.

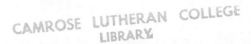

III. Aging Processes
   A. Health depends on the vitality and health of the cells.
   B. Biological age (which is not related to chronological age) is measured by changes in the structure and functioning of the major body systems.
   C. The biological-aging process can be accelerated by factors which can lead to deterioration of the body, disease, and premature death (death prior to estimations for the general population).
   D. Exercise physiologists have shown that physical exercise, if sufficiently intensive, can delay the phenomena of aging.

IV. Degenerative Body Conditions
   A. The first signs of degenerative body conditions usually appear as premature damage to the cardiovascular and respiratory systems.
   B. The Respiratory System and Breathing
      1. The respiratory system contains the organs in which oxygen and carbon dioxide are exchanged.
      2. Exercise conditions the muscles of the rib cage and diaphragm.
         a. When an active person inhales, the muscles must create a large vacuum into which the lungs expand.
         b. When an active person exhales, the muscles must recoil and squeeze back into a smaller area.
      3. During the aging process, there is a normal decrease in the gas-exchange capabilities of a person's lungs.
         a. This is largely responsible for the decreasing physical ability of advancing age.
         b. Adequate physical activity can delay this biological-aging process.
      4. The amount of air which a person can process in a specific amount of time is a signficant indicator of his physical condition. Any deterioration of the lung tissues reduces the capability of the lungs to process air.
      5. Insufficient activity, air pollution, irritations, and disease organisms can decrease the effectiveness of the lungs to the point where specific symptoms of certain diseases appear.
      6. Emphysema is a degenerative condition in which the lung tissues lose their elasticity and the walls of the alveoli break down.
      7. Bronchitis is a condition caused by an inflamed and infected lining of the bronchial tubes. Bronchitis often leads to emphysema.

C. The Cardiovascular System and Circulation
1. From the lungs, oxygen goes directly into the bloodstream.
2. The factors in the blood which affect health include the following:
   a. The number of red blood cells.
   b. The amount of hemoglobin in the red blood cells.
3. A totally fit individual has a larger blood supply than an average man of comparable size.
   a. He has more hemoglobin.
   b. He has more blood plasma (the fluid portion of the blood).
   c. He has more total blood volume.
4. The heart takes oxygen-filled blood from the lungs and pumps it throughout the body. It also takes carbon-dioxide-filled blood from the body and pumps it into the lungs.
   a. The heart works harder, faster, and less efficiently in a nonexerciser than in a totally fit individual.
   b. The heart of a totally fit person can beat less because the decreased heart rate is more than compensated for by increased blood volume.
5. As the volume of blood increases, the body builds more blood vessels.
6. In the totally fit individual, blood pressure is usually lower than in the nonexerciser. Reduced blood pressure is retained only as long as one remains in condition.
7. Coronary heart disease—one of the major causes of atherosclerosis is lack of exercise.
8. Lifetime muscular activity will lead to a decrease in the incidence of degenerative cardiovascular conditions.
V. Total Fitness and Muscular Activity
   A. Exercise and the Skeletal Muscles
   1. There are different kinds of exercises and activities which affect these muscles.
      a. Some are aimed at building, or enlarging, skeletal muscles.
      b. Bicycling, running, jogging, swimming, and tennis contribute to total fitness.
   2. Sports contributing to total fitness result in two important changes:
      a. The muscles grow longer and leaner so more of the cells are closer to the blood vessels.
      b. New blood vessels are produced.
   3. The building of muscles up to the point where a person can perform in a total fitness program is the value of muscle-strengthening exercises.

B. Exercise and the Smooth Muscles
1. Physical conditioning increases the elasticity of the muscles and their ability to contract.
2. Exercise improves the performance of the smooth muscles.

VI. Body Flexibility
A. Flexibility—the ability to move freely in various directions—involves a wide range of body motions.
B. Good body flexibility permits greater freedom of body movements and helps prevent muscle injuries.
C. A total fitness program improves flexibility because muscles, ligaments, and connecting tissues are repeatedly stretched.

VII. Body Coordination
A. A coordinated person is able to use the proper muscles with proper force at the proper time.
B. The most significant point in coordination development is that muscular activity increases an individual's ability to perform more muscular activity.

VIII. Mental Values of Total Fitness
A. Physical activity enables the whole body to operate efficiently and to withstand the stresses imposed on it.
B. Proprioception ("muscle sense") provides the mind with its understanding of stretch, tension, movement, body position, and the third dimension.
C. Every movement, every body position, and every tension in a muscle, tendon, and joint help to contribute to the formation of concepts and ideas.
D. Competitive sports are an important stimulus to the body; the muscles must perform efficiently, and the mind must make quick, accurate decisions while maintaining control over the emotions.

IX. Resistance to Communicable Diseases
A. Physical exercise increases body resistance to oxygen debt, overheating, and chilling.
B. Physical exercise also increases resistance to some poisons.
C. Processes important to the control of disease operate more efficiently in the trained individual than they do in the untrained individual.

X. Most physical activity improves and promotes the efficiency of the whole organism and is essential to the proper functioning and maintenance of all systems of the body.

QUESTIONS FOR REVIEW

1. Define growth. What is the relationship between growth and physical activity?

2. Explain biological age. Contrast it with chronological age.
3. What are the relationships between biological age and total fitness?
4. Define premature death.
5. What are the relationships between the aging processes and the respiratory system?
6. Explain the significant diseases of the respiratory system which are linked to aging and degeneration.
7. Describe the factors which limit an individual's ability to perform when he is not in condition.

Chapter 5
ACTIVITY
FOR ALL AGES

In 1965 the President's Council on Physical Fitness and Sports recommended daily classes in physical education for all grade-school pupils. Physical education is important because it supplies children's needs for exercise while it contributes to physical development and lays the foundation for exercise habits in later years. If, from a young age, children are taught the principles of physical fitness discussed in the first three chapters of this book, they will grow into adults inclined to participate in vigorous physical activity.

While he is in high school and college, an individual should develop skills in several different activities in which to participate throughout his life. In planning activities which will continue throughout life, three factors should be considered. Physical activities should develop muscular strength, muscular endurance, and circulatory endurance. All activities which improve or maintain total fitness must involve these basic activities: vigorous running, lifting of body weight, and quick changes in direction. They should also provide the individual with knowledge of ways to maintain and further develop strength and endurance.

All physical activity involves work, but physical activity can be pleasant as well. Enjoyable activities are usually ones which are not closely identified with exercise programs or with work. Exercise programs often seem tedious because goals can be reached only in the distant future and improvements are not immediately visible. A common problem with today's well-publicized physical fitness programs is that they are boring.

Since regular participation in an activity depends on enthusiasm and motivation, a person should choose activities he enjoys. If an activity is not enjoyable, a person will stop participating in it.

The best way to exercise is to participate in a demanding sport which provides immediate satisfaction. Individual and dual sports such as tennis, badminton, handball, swimming, skiing, and bicycling are examples of such "fun" or "play" sports. Activities such as running and jogging provide a faster workout but require more dedication because they do not have the built-in motivation of sports.

People are more easily motivated to participate in sports than in other physical activities and are more likely to continue participating in them throughout life. Even the most beneficial of sports will not, however, produce significant results unless they are vigorously pursued during participation.

POSTURE

No one can avoid all physical activities. Posture, holding the body erect against the force of gravity, is a form of exercise. Posture is the way you normally, and unconsciously, control your body when you are standing (presumably straight and relaxed), sitting, walking, running, and engaging in any other physical activity.

Walking posture is called *carriage*, running posture *gait*, and athletic posture *form*. All involve the same principle: management of the muscles in order to overcome the force of gravity with ease. Good posture and body control are natural, not forced.

Fitness is a necessity for proper posture, since posture depends on the ability of muscles to respond. Physical exercise increases the tone of your muscles and helps them respond to the unconscious commands that maintain proper posture. An individual does not maintain perfect posture all of the time. However, he should be able to maintain it comfortably, whenever necessary.

Standing Posture

Standing posture is not forced; it is a way of balancing the body. A graceful and efficient person has proper posture. The failure of clothes to drape and hang properly is often caused by faulty standing posture. Correction of faulty posture does much for the figure, or body build.

When standing, imagine that your body consists of three separate areas, the head, the upper torso, and the lower torso, which are balanced on two points, the balls of the feet. Unless the head, upper torso, and lower torso are in line with one another, your standing posture will be strained and abnormal. In a properly balanced body, an imaginary straight line drawn through the body should pass through the lobe of the ear and the bump of the anklebone.

The single most important suggestion for obtaining good standing posture is to "stand tall." An excellent exercise to help you to maintain standing posture is to stand with your back to a wall or door. Your head, buttocks, and heels should touch the surface of the wall. Stretch your hands out over your head along the wall. Now elevate yourself on your toes. Repeat this six to twelve times. If done periodically, this exercise will give you the feeling of proper balance and will help you obtain the muscle coordination needed for proper standing posture.

Sitting Posture (Reclining Posture)

When you are sitting, reclining, or lying down, good posture is any body position which is comfortable to you over a period of time. At rest the body moves freely and frequently to rest groups of slightly fatigued muscles.

However, when you must sit upright to eat, work at a desk, or engage in conversation, you will find that you are more comfortable and far less fatigued if you sit properly. Here again, balance your body as you did for standing posture. Balance your head and shoulders (upper torso) directly over your hips (lower torso). To do this plant your feet firmly on the floor; sit back on the seat of the chair comfortably erect, balancing your head over your hips. Whenever you reach forward in this position, roll forward from your hips; don't simply reach out with your arms. If you practice sitting properly and rocking forward a few times, you will find a natural, comfortable posture whenever you sit.

Walking Posture (Carriage)

The sense of balance is activated by body movements. Consequently, people usually walk more properly than they sit or stand. Balancing the body over the balls of the feet will insure the proper balance needed for walking. This balance is maintained without voluntary effort. To achieve a natural way of walking, let your thigh lead your body. If you first contract the muscles which lift the thigh, you can walk without effort. Walk naturally, stride from the hip, lift the thighs, and be as comfortable as possible.

When you are walking, the distance between your feet should be about the same as it is when you are standing comfortably. To improve your carriage, practice walking a straight line (the edge of a carpet or a line of tiles). This exercise will teach you not to toe out and not to walk with your feet too far apart.

High-heeled shoes can cause special posture problems. They place excessive strain on the ankles and on the arches of the feet and, thus, cause the body to be thrown out of balance. When wearing high-heeled shoes, women should make a special effort to balance or they will walk incorrectly. For daily use, heels should not be more than one and one-half inches high, and the base of the heel should be nearly as broad as the top. Because high, narrow heels make the ankles roll, they may cause injuries and permanent damage. Women with strong arches can safely wear high heels if the heels are not too high and too narrow and if they are not worn too frequently. Women with weak arches or poor posture should not wear high heels until they have strengthened their arches and improved their posture.

FATIGUE

When a muscle is stimulated beyond its ability to recover, it will refuse to respond (page 17). The muscle's inability to contract is called muscle fatigue. Muscle fatigue is localized; it occurs in one muscle or in one group of muscles. General body fatigue is much greater in scope and must be considered from a different viewpoint. It is related to work load, total fitness, accumulation of cellular wastes, and depletion of body sugar. This kind of fatigue is called *physical fatigue.*

Physical exercise should produce some degree of physical fatigue. Undue fatigue, however, is damaging. A person should get enough exercise and physiological stress to bring him to, but not beyond, the fatigue point. An individual's point of undue fatigue depends on his ability to accommodate stress of both a physical and an emotional nature, for physical fatigue may be caused by emotional, as well as physical, factors. In fact, in modern society, with all of its laborsaving devices and appliances, muscular fatigue has almost been eliminated, and emotional and mental fatigue have taken its place.

General body functioning is a continual response to various internal and external stresses. Stressful situations, whether they are physical or emotional, produce various physiological reactions. In 1956

Hans Selye, a Canadian endocrinologist, reported that regardless of the form of stress, the body's response is always the same. Selye called this response the *stress syndrome,* or *general adaptation syndrome* (GAS).

Changes brought about by stress may eventually cause degenerative conditions such as ulcers of the digestive tract, high blood pressure, heart conditions, and asthmatic reactions. These diseases result from local reactions to total body stress. In *Physiology of Exercise,* Herbert A. de Vries states, "Humans seldom die of old age; they die because of weakness or uneven wear of one organ or system."

Body reactions to stress occur in three stages:

1. the alarm reaction
2. the stage of resistance
3. the stage of exhaustion

The period of alarm reaction is the period in which the symptoms of the general adaption syndrome (undue fatigue or symptoms of a specific disease) appear. If the stress is of long duration, the individual enters the stage of resistance during which the stress syndrome seems to disappear, and the resistance of the individual is greater. Everyone inherits a certain amount of resistance to stress. Selye called this resistance *adaptational energy.* Evidence indicates that physical fitness increases an individual's adaptational energy. Consequently, totally fit individuals are much more able to control and accommodate stress and fatigue than are passively fit individuals. Finally, if the adaptation energy is overcome by stress, the stage of exhaustion is entered, the general adaptation syndrome reappears, and death from exhaustion may eventually occur.

Competitive athletes are trained and conditioned to push themselves far beyond their normal fatigue points. This is dangerous if done without medical advice and guidance by experts on physical education. In competitive training programs an individual's adaptation energy is of major importance. A competitive event is more stressful (emotionally and physically) and, thus, more fatiguing than a training session. A person's overall stress load regulates his adaptation energy. During training a two-thirds maximum load will maintain peak conditioning. Overload intervals of short duration increase conditioning, but when prolonged, such overloading may lead to fatigue and a loss of peak conditioning.

Table 5.1 shows the relationships between each of the three phases of Selye's general adaptation syndrome and the phases involved in an athlete's training.

Exhaustion, or loss of adaptational energy, can occur in any person who tries to push himself beyond his current physical capacities. Unfortunately, former high school and college athletes and overly enthusiastic beginners sometimes try to do this. They may try to crowd

Table 5.1   Relationships Between GAS and Phases of Training

PHASES OF GAS	PHASES OF TRAINING
1. Alarm reaction stage	1. Phase of adaptation: time in which fundamental training is initiated and progresses toward peak performance (five to twelve weeks)
2. Resistance stage	2. Completed adaptation: achievement of peak condition (three to six weeks)
3. Exhaustion stage	3. Readaptation: loss of peak condition or overtraining (starts six to sixteen weeks after beginning of training)

a year's exercise into a weekend of skiing or a week's exercise into an afternoon of football. For people who are under thirty years old and who do not lead completely passive lives, the result of undue fatigue is stiffness and soreness. For people who are older and who are only passively fit, the result may be a serious stroke, a heart atack, or death.

The amount of exercise a person should undertake depends on his age and his physical condition. Athletes need more exercise than the average adult. Youngsters need more exercise than adults because their activities are much more vigorous. A physical peak of muscular strength, coordination, and body activity occurs in the early twenties. This seems to be true of most physical and physiological activities of the body. As a system, the body seems to reach its peak when a person is about twenty-two years old. This is why so many norms in physiology (weight, respiration, blood pressure, etc.) are calculated for the ages twenty to twenty-five. Age is a critical factor in both the choice of exercise and the amount of exercise a person can perform.

Unless he has kept himself in training for competitive sports, a person who is over thirty should not participate in vigorous competitive activities or in endurance exercises without prior conditioning. Fortunately, the body has a built-in signal to warn against overexercise —pain! This signal should be heeded rather than ignored in the excitment of the moment. When engaging in any physical exercise, a person should always pay attention to any pain, mild or severe, that the exercise causes. When he feels pain, he should rest. Only rest will overcome fatigue.

As you have seen, exercise builds resistance to fatigue. However, the manner of rewarding the body is as effective in allaying fatigue as the reward itself. In other words, fatigue is most easily avoided if a parson derives satisfaction and pleasure from physical activities. If the activities are repetitive or dull, the process of obtaining exercise will itself cause fatigue.

Exercise is, of course, only one aspect of fitness. The value of exercise may be overrated, as well as underrated. To be totally fit, a person must also have adequate nutrition, sufficient rest, and activies which stimulate his mind.

THE EFFECTS OF SLEEP

Muscular rest or a change in muscular activities can alleviate fatigue. However, the body cannot continue to function only on rest or activity change; eventually, it must have sleep. During sleep the body is never completely relaxed. It constantly changes positions, even during periods of deep sleep. One reason for this is that circulation must reach tissues on which the body is exerting pressure. If body movements did not occur, tissues would die from lack of oxygen.

Sleep is a temporary state of unconsciousness during which voluntary thinking is suspended, muscular activity is greatly reduced, and blood pressure, pulse, and body temperature rates are also reduced. These rate decreases are signs of the need for sleep, and they reach their minimum levels in the first two hours of sleep. About an hour before a person wakes, his body systems begin to accelerate toward the levels maintained during wakefulness.

An important biological pattern is a person's pattern of sleep and wakefulness. Even if a person were to remain in total darkness or in total light, he would still maintain approximately the same sleep-wakefulness pattern.

Studies of the brain indicate that while a person is awake, numerous nerve impulses pass continuously throughout the brain. The degree of wakefulness seems to be related to the amount of impulse activity occurring in the brain. When the impulse activity decreases, a person relaxes, becomes drowsy, and, at a certain point, falls asleep. Sleep is caused and maintained by a significant decrease in neural activity.

Wakefulness is maintained by a continuous transmission of nervous impulses to the muscles and to the autonomic nervous system (the system which regulates the functioning of the internal organs). A high degree of wakefulness increases the tone of all muscles, giving a person the feeling of muscular readiness. The stimulation of the sympathetic nervous system increases the rate of metabolism, and, thus, enables the body to perform increased amounts of exercise. Such increased neuromuscular activity periodically fatigues the synapses (the junctions between nerve cells) of the central nervous system, reducing the transmission of neural impulses. The reduction of impulses permits selective areas of the brain to become dormant; this is sleep.

The nervous system seems to slump into neurofatigue shortly before a person falls asleep, and it shows signs of being rested at the termination of sleep. Sleep has many effects. It seems to have a greater effect on neurological and emotional aspects of physical fatigue than on pure physical fatigue. Sleep conserves the energies of most parts of the body. Sleep also reestablishes the balance of excitability among the different parts of the central nervous system. As a person becomes fatigued, some areas of the central nervous system lose excitability more rapidly than others. This is evident in the actions of different individuals as they fatigue. Extreme fatigue can precipitate extreme psychotic reactions. After prolonged sleep, inappropriate actions and feelings are relieved, and the proper degrees of excitability and control are reestablished.

Excess muscular fatigue, caused by prolonged, vigorous physical activity, is not conducive to sound, pleasurable sleep. Moderate exercise is helpful in promoting sleep. It seems to relieve muscular and emotional tensions. This induces a state of relaxation which provides the optimum conditions for sleep. When a person is asleep, his muscles are more relaxed than they are when he is awake, but they are never completely relaxed. An individual's ability to relax his muscles is one of the secrets of falling asleep. Dr. Edmund Jacobson[1] created the following series of exercises which are conducive to sleep. If you try these relaxing exercises, do them after you have found a comfortable position in bed.

1. Clench your fists tightly enough to feel tautness in your muscles. Then open and relax your hands on the bed.

2. Tense and relax your arm muscles until you feel your muscles relaxing.

3. Now start relaxing your muscles by letting the parts go limp, beginning with your toes and working toward your head: toes, feet, lower leg, upper leg, thigh, trunk, mouth, forehead, and eyelids. By the time you reach the eyelids, you should fall asleep.

How Much Sleep Is Needed?

The amount of sleep a person needs is influenced by his rate of metabolism and his body growth. Rapidly growing infants need more sleep than children do, and children need more than adults. People who are not very active often need more sleep than do active people. People recovering from an illness may need an increased amount of sleep.

A person's ability to sleep is affected by several factors:

1. *Prior amount of sleep.*   Length of sleep the previous night and duration of naps or rest periods during the day.

[1]Edmund Jacobson, M.D., *You Must Relax*, Revised Edition (New York, Whittlesey House, 1942).

2. *Anxiety.* The tensions of the day grea\
night's sleep.

3. *Daily problems.* The overall emotional h\
dividual influences his sleep patterns.

4. *Degree and amount of physical exertion.*
above, mild exercise promotes sleep; vigorous exercise ofte

5. *Attitudes.* An individual's cultural background ...d habits
influence his sleep patterns.

The test of whether or not an individual is getting enough
sleep is a simple, practical one. It consists of one question: How do
you feel in the morning? A person is getting enough sleep if he wakes
up in the morning refreshed and ready for the day. In applying this
test, discount the first half hour of wakefulness because there are variations in the length of time it takes for people's neuromuscular activity
to rise to a level of full wakefulness.

PRINCIPLES OF EXERCISE PROGRAMS

Although the concepts of exercise have changed drastically in
recent years, the principles have not changed. Modern total fitness programs are the result of laboratory studies that have added greatly to
our knowledge. Exercise is now considered essential to counterbalance
today's sedentary life styles.

In choosing a program, people often ask, "How much and
what kind of exercise do I need?" In *The New Aerobics,* Dr. Kenneth
H. Cooper points out that the body needs both oxygen and the rhythmic
physical activity which supplies the body with oxygen. During exercise, the blood is richer in oxygen and nutrients and more effectively
eliminates wastes from muscles and other organs. Activities which promote efficient body functioning include walking, running, swimming,
bicycling, dancing, skiing, and tennis. Also, if exercise is to be effective,
it must be performed regularly and at one's capacity.

If you are satisfied with your ability to function at your present level, all you need to do is exercise to maintain this level. However,
if you are dissatisfied with your physical condition and want to improve
it, you should take several steps before you start a total fitness program.

1. Have a complete medical examination, especially if you
are over thirty years of age. No one over thirty should start on any
total fitness program without first consulting a physician. Part of your
medical examination should be an exercise capacity test (bicycle ergom-
eter or treadmill test).

2. Have your program planned by a competent exercise
physiologist or physical education specialist.

Any total fitness program should include exercises which develop or maintain the three requirements of physical fitness: muscular strength, muscular endurance, and circulatory endurance.

Muscular Strength and Muscular Endurance

Muscular strength is the maximum amount of force, or tension, a muscle can exert in a single contraction. Muscles develop strength when they are subjected to tension in progressively increasing amounts. Muscular endurance is the ability of the muscles either to maintain a maximum contraction or to respond repetitively for a relatively long time. Before he undertakes any total fitness activities, an individual must possess sufficient strength to support his body weight easily throughout the activity. Two types of muscular contractions, isometric contractions and isotonic contractions, may be used to develop muscular strength and endurance.

Isometric contractions are produced by pushing or pulling against an immovable object. When held for a long period of time, they tension produce, or static contractions. Such "dynamic tension" exercise programs began to gain popularity in the late 1930s because of a vigorous advertising campaign which appealed to young men interested in developing muscular physiques. The person who designed the isometric program called "Dynamic Tension" was Charles Atlas.

The systematic isometric contraction of the muscles of the body will, within days, improve muscular strength, provided the program is of sufficient time durations. Best results appear to be obtained by using maximal contraction strength, held for 5 to 8 seconds and repeated five to ten times daily. Care must be taken to exercise opposing muscle groups at equal strength or unequal strength patterns will develop. Also, isometric exercises do not develop muscular endurance or flexibility. These exercises develop large muscles which can produce great muscle tension during isometric contractions. Sustained for longer periods of time (over 8 seconds), such contractions produce a rapid rise in blood pressure; in one minute mean blood pressure can rise as far as 140.

Isometric contractions are also produced when people move or lift extremely heavy loads—when, for example, they open a window which is stuck or shovel snow (a common cause of heart attacks). Isometric contractions occur, too, when overweight individuals try to do push-ups or pull-ups. A reasonably fit person may use 30 percent of his muscle power to do a push-up while someone 20 pounds overweight uses 40 percent of his muscle power to do the same thing. Blood pressure rate rises in response to the intensity of the tension and the length of time it is held. Therefore, untrained, older, or overweight persons should not use isometrics, move heavy objects, or become overly tense. The high blood pressures produced may be very dangerous to them.

The size of the muscle group in use seems to have nothing to do with increases in blood pressure. Small muscles in the back of the neck which become overly tense because of nerves or fatigue produce a rise in blood pressure equivalent to that produced by large leg muscles pushing against a stationary object.

Isotonic contractions are produced when an individual continues to raise, lower, or move a moderate load. Within isotonic exercise programs it is possible to do many combinations of *repetitions*[2] (the total number of executions), *resistance* (weight to be lifted), and *sets* (the number of groups of repetitions done consecutively without resting).

Muscular strength is best developed when the resistance is relatively high and the number of repetitions is low. Muscular endurance is best developed when the resistance is relatively low and the number of repetitions is high. For example, in weight training, muscular strength is most successfully developed by lifting a selected weight only six times; muscular endurance, flexibility, and coordination are better served by selecting a lighter weight and lifting it fifteen to twenty times.

Resistance may be applied in different ways. Because body weight is considered to be resistance, isotonic contractions are produced whenever someone moves. Calisthenics and weight training are good ways to apply resistance, especially for people who start a total fitness program after a period of sedentary living. Isotonic programs are most successful in developing strength and endurance if they are performed prior to and during an organized fitness training program.

Isotonic programs have several advantages. First, the exercises may be systematically planned to cover all muscle groups of the body and to emphasize areas of greatest need. Also, it is easy to adjust the degree of exercise from very mild forms to vigorous efforts. Finally, the exercises may be performed easily in the home. Many activities producing isotonic contractions will occur to the person seeking variety and interest in activities designed to develop adequate muscular strength and endurance.

Circulatory Endurance

Exercises for circulatory endurance stimulate an increase in cardiorespiratory functioning, producing results known as conditioning, training effect, and aerobic capacity. Essentially, such exercises

[2]In many exercise programs the word "repetition" is used incorrectly. *Execution maximum* (EM) or *repetition maximum* (RM) should be used to indicate repetitions. Both terms indicate the maximum weight that can be lifted for an indicated number of repetitions. For example, 10 EM (RM) is the greatest weight that can be lifted ten times.

involve isotonic activities which are continued over a period of time (a minimum of 15 minutes) and at a pace necessary to increase the pulse rate to between 130 and 132 beats per minute during the exercise. In addition to circulatory endurance, these activities produce flexibility and coordination.

During long periods of sustained activity, heavy demands are made on the lungs and the circulatory system, including the heart. Improved circulatory endurance results in increases in the oxygen-carrying ability of the blood, the number of the capillaries, and cardiac efficiency and output.

Isometric exercises develop strength but usually do not improve circulatory endurance. However, if the repetitions of weight training are done rapidly and are continued until a person is perspiring and breathing heavily (pulse rate is nearing 132), they may be helpful to circulatory endurance. Furthermore, isometric exercises may be performed in conjunction with jogging, hopping, or running in place.

Individual sports such as hiking, brisk walking, jogging, skipping, skating, running, cross-country skiing, bicycling, and swimming are particularly good for circulatory endurance. Distance, speed, and duration may be regulated to the capability of the individual. Progression in the amount of exercise may be planned from day to day. Other sports have a potentially good effect on circulatory endurance. Among these are the dual sports handball, squash, and tennis, and the team sports soccer, basketball, and ice hockey.

Exercise Tolerance

Exercise tolerance is the level at which the body responds favorably to exercise. An individual's exercise tolerance is his ability to perform a series of exercises, participate in a sport, or enjoy a walk without undue fatigue. All exercises should be adapted to an individual's tolerance level. Activities which are too easy for someone fall short of his tolerance, while exercises that are too difficult or are impossible should not be attempted.

One indication of exercise tolerance is pulse rate. Exercise physiologists have found that if a person works at 60 percent of his capacity, his body undergoes favorable circulatory changes which lead to a trained, or fit, condition. People under thirty years of age work at 60 percent of their capacity when their pulse rate is 151 beats per minute. People over thirty work at 60 percent of their capacity when their pulse reaches 131 beats per minute. The decreased work capacity of people over thirty is caused partly by the decrease in heart rate which comes with advancing age and partly by the reduced elasticity of the blood vessels.

A person who performs calisthenics, lifts weights, or participates in an individual or dual sport can monitor his own pulse rate.

To do this he should take his pulse rate for ten seconds immediately after he stops exercising. He may then multiply the ten-second rate by six to obtain his rate per minute. If he is over thirty and his pulse rate is 22 x 6, or 132 beats per minute, he has worked adequately but has not overexercised.

If a person engages in four periods of exercise each week and in each period works at 60 per cent of his work load capacity for 15 minutes, he can maintain his body in a trained condition. Of course, not all people should work at 60 percent of their capacity. People with cardiovascular conditions, for example, should not elevate their pulse rates to 131 beats per minute. Before beginning any exercise program, a person should consult his physician; once in a program, he should continue to have periodic physical examinations. He should also consult a competent physical educator for instruction in individual and dual sports and for advice on the best exercise program for him.

Overloading and Progression

The body has great ability to adapt to stress. Therefore, people who wish to improve their performance and their general condition should continually increase the duration and intensity of their exercises. The process of extending oneself beyond usual physical effort is called *overloading*, or, more recently, *interval training*. Harder work with less energy output may be accomplished by overloading. Overloading involves gradually increasing stress, in terms of the following factors:

1. Gradually and progressively increasing the speed of performance.

2. Gradually increasing the total load (resistance).

3. Progressively increasing the total time that a given position can be held.

4. Maintaining a constant resistance and progressively increasing the total number of repetitions.

In exercises designed to develop strength or circulatory endurance, intervals of overloading should be of extremely short duration (15 or 20 seconds) and should be kept within one's tolerance level. Fatigue may be delayed by reducing the work load, by slowing the rhythm, and by breathing regularly and deeply. In using interval training, a person may alternately run and walk to give himself periods to recover from stress.

The principles of overloading should help you increase your efficiency and performance. As you master an exercise program you should progress to more strenuous exercises.

Progression is accomplished when increments of work, or sets, are added at appropriate steps. All exercise plans should provide for progression. Generally, increasing the intensity, or the tempo, of an exercise is more important than increasing its duration. Through progression, people begin with easy exercises and work toward more and more difficult ones.

Warming Up

In the way that an athlete must train to reach the level of physical fitness at which he can perform safely, a nonathlete must also take time to develop the strength, coordination, and endurance demanded by any sport. When individuals have not exercised on a regular basis for a number of years, they should recondition themselves on a warm-up basis. Too often, sedentary people who exercise become sore or injured because their muscles and joints are not ready for activity. A warm-up program of 15 to 20 minutes followed by slow walking and jogging will help prevent soreness and muscle injury. Such a program should be followed until the body is reconditioned enough to withstand more vigorous exercise. An individual should allow a minimum of one month of reconditioning for each year he has been out of condition.

Also, each time a person exercises or participates in a sport, he should first warm up. A proper warm-up prepares a person for exercise by increasing body temperature, stretching ligaments, and slightly increasing cardiovascular activity. The amount of warm-up necessary varies among individuals and generally increases with age.

You should begin at a very slow pace with light, rhythmical exercises, accompanied by stretching and deep breathing. Deep breathing before exercising temporarily increases your oxygen supply and will help you to take deeper breaths while exercising. A simple deep-breathing exercise is shown in Figure 5.1. The next activity should be a series of exercises to stretch and loosen the muscles and raise the heartbeat and body temperature enough to promote sweating (Figures 5.2, 5.3, 5.4).

The end of the warm-up session is an excellent time to exercise the feet. Too often, extreme damage is done to the feet because of neglect. All sports and exercises depend on the feet. Spend the last five minutes of your warm-up following this set of foot exercises:

First Exercise.   Drop a dozen marbles on the floor. Sit down and pick them up one by one with the toes of one foot; then drop them into a container. Repeat the procedure with the other foot.

Second Exercise.   Sit down on the floor and cross one leg over the other at the knee. Take hold of the toes of the top leg with both hands. Then try to curl your toes as hard as you can while resisting the pressure with your hands. Repeat the procedure with the other foot.

Third Exercise.   Sit on the floor with one leg flexed at the knee and the foot flat on the floor. Extend the other leg, raise the foot off the floor, point the toes, and make a full circle with the foot. Repeat this ten times with each foot.

Fourth Exercise. Stand with your hands on your hips. Rise up on tiptoe, hold it, then drop to the floor. Repeat ten times at the beginning, and build up to twenty or more times for each warm-up session.

Easing Off

Just as the body needs warming up, it also needs easing off after exercise. This helps return the blood to the heart and the body temperature back to normal. You should keep moving for several minutes after vigorous activity until your breathing has returned to normal, the stress of the exercise has subsided, and the body has cooled.

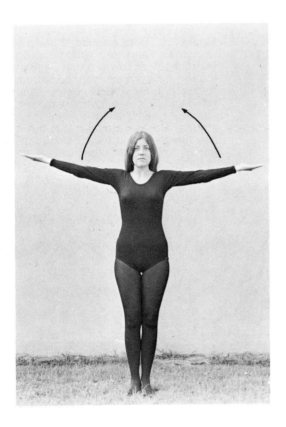
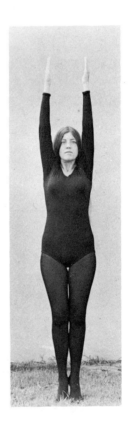

Figure 5.1 Deep breathing exercise. Stand tall; rise on your tiptoes, and inhale deeply. As you inhale and rise, raise your arms in half circles until your hands come together over your head. Hold this extended position for 1 or 2 minutes. Then lower your arms and drop back to the standing position as you exhale (six to twelve breaths are sufficient).

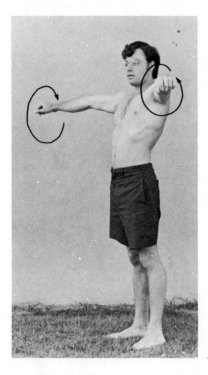

Figure 5.2 Arm rotation. Extend your arms straight out from the shoulders, and rotate them so that your hands are tracing circles about 1 foot in diameter. Do twenty circles rotating forward, and twenty circles rotating backward.

Figure 5.3 Body rotation. With your legs wide apart and your hand on your hips, lean forward and bend at the waist. Now rotate your body from the waist in great, slow circles. Lean far enough to the right, rear, left, and front so you feel the muscles stretch. Do five circles, rotating in one direction, and five circles rotating in the other direction.

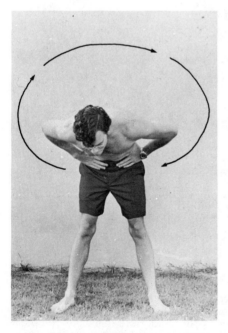

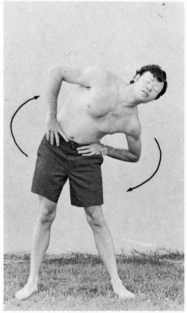

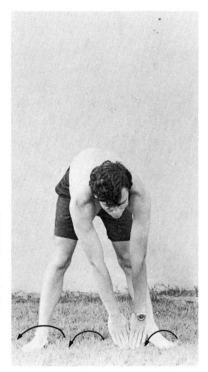

Figure 5.4 Bend and bounce. With your legs spread apart, bend down and touch your fingers to the ground outside of your right foot. Repeat the three bounces with the left foot. If you are just beginning a conditioning program, do not, at first, try to touch the ground, and do not bounce. Bend enough to feel the back muscles stretch; each day, increase the tension on the muscles until you have regained your flexibility.

TOTAL FITNESS CONDITIONING

The three principles of physical fitness (muscular strength, muscular endurance, and circulatory endurance) should be incorporated into any total fitness program. Exercise alone, however, does not guarantee fitness. The American Medical Association has stated that sufficient rest and sleep, an adequate diet, and regular exercise are all necessary for total body fitness.

The minimum exercise recommendations are from 30 to 60 minutes every other day. For a total fitness program to be effective, exercise should be regular. However, the value of exercise depends more on how it is done than on how often it is done. Exercise must be vigorous enough to raise the pulse beat to 131 beats per minute for people over thirty and 151 for people under thirty; increased pulse beat should be sustained for at least 15 minutes. A five-hour game of golf over eighteen holes won't do this for anyone. This is the reason why popular sports such as golf and bowling should be supplemented by an exercise program.

To follow a daily exercise program, use a combination of programs consisting of interval training and change of pace. Change of pace includes one or both of the following:

1. The shifting from one activity to another which involves a different set of muscles and a different kind of exercise.

2. The changing of the intensity of exercise.

The time of day that you exercise depends on your schedule and your preferences. Some people enjoy an early morning workout; others like to exercise after a day's work. Individual exercise programs must subject stress to the body within the limits of a person's exercise tolerance. The body will develop to meet the demands placed on it, and overloading and progression should be employed as tolerance extends. Each exercise program session should be started by warming up and ended by easing off.

SUMMARY

    I. Physical education should supply the individual's immediate needs for exercise while it contributes to physical development and lays the foundation for exercise habits in later years.

   II. While he is in high school and college, an individual should develop skill in several activities in which to participate throughout life. Physical activities should develop
       A. Muscular strength.
       B. Muscular endurance.
       C. Circulatory endurance.

 III. Posture is the way a person normally and unconsciously controls his body when he is standing, sitting, walking, running, and engaging in any other physical activity.
       A. Standing Posture
          1. Standing posture is not forced; it is a way of balancing the body.
          2. The head, upper torso, and lower torso should be in line with one another.
       B. Sitting Posture
          1. Any body position which is comfortable over a period of time.
          2. To eat and to work, sit upright with the body balanced as it is for standing posture.
       C. Walking Posture (Carriage)
          1. Let your thigh lead the body.
          2. Balance your body over the balls of the feet.
       D. General Posture Problems
          1. Positioning
          2. Fatigue

 IV. Fatigue
       A. Muscular fatigue (the inability of a muscle to contract) is localized; it occurs in one muscle or in one group of muscles.

B. General Body Fatigue (Physical Fatigue)
  1. Related to work load, total fitness, accumulation of cellular wastes, and depletion of body sugar.
  2. Physical fatigue can be caused by emotional, as well as physical, factors. In fact, modern society has substituted emotional psychological fatigue for muscular fatigue.
  3. General body functioning is a continual response to various internal and external stresses.
     a. The body's response to stress is called general adaptation syndrome (GAS).
        (1) alarm reaction
        (2) stage of resistance
        (3) stage of exhaustion
     b. Totally fit individuals are more able to control stress and, thus, fatigue than are unfit individuals.
V. The Effects of Sleep
  A. Muscular rest or a change in muscular activities can alleviate fatigue; however, the body cannot continue to function without sleep.
  B. Excess muscular fatigue is not conducive to sound pleasurable sleep. Moderate exercise is helpful in promoting sleep.
  C. How much sleep is needed? Do you wake up in the morning refreshed and ready for the day?
VI. Principles of Exercise Programs
  A. Although the concepts of exercise have changed drastically in recent years, the principles have not changed.
  B. If exercise is to be effective, it must be performed regularly and at one's capacity.
  C. A person should take several steps before beginning an exercise program:
    1. He should have a complete medical examination, including an exercise capacity test.
    2. He should have his program planned by an exercise physiologist or a physical education specialist.
  D. Any total fitness program should include exercises which develop or maintain the three requirements of physical fitness: muscular strength, muscular endurance, and circulatory endurance.
    1. Muscular Strength and Muscular Endurance
       a. Muscular strength is the maximum amount of force, or tension, a muscle can exert in a single contraction.
       b. Muscular endurance is the ability of the muscles either to maintain a maximum contraction or to respond repetitively for a relatively long time.

        c. Isometric contractions produce muscle strength.

        d. Isotonic contractions produce both muscle strength and endurance.

    2. Circulatory endurance is cardiorespiratory functioning which produces results called conditioning, training effect, and aerobic capacity.

        a. Improved circulatory endurance results in an increase in the oxygen-carrying ability of the blood, the number or the involvement of the capillaries, and cardiac efficiency and output.

        b. Exercises which improve circulatory endurance also produce flexibility and coordination.

 E. Exercise Tolerance

    1. The level at which the body responds to exercise favorably.

        a. Pulse rate of 151 for individuals under thirty years of age.

        b. Pulse rate of 131 for individuals over thirty years of age.

    2. Any exercise should be adapted to each individual's tolerance level.

 F. Overloading and Progression

    1. Overloading is the process of extending oneself beyond usual physical effort.

    2. Progression is a gradual increase in complexity of exercises.

 G. Warming Up

    1. Individuals who have not exercised regularly for a number of years should recondition themselves on a warm-up basis.

    2. Each time one exercises or participates in a sport, he should first warm up.

VII. Total Fitness Conditioning

 A. It should always include the three principles of physical fitness (muscular strength, muscular endurance, and circulatory endurance).

 B. It should be performed regularly.

 C. It should consist of interval training and change of pace.

QUESTIONS FOR REVIEW

1. Total fitness activities should develop what three principles?
2. There are two definitions of warming up. Explain these two definitions. How are they related?
3. Define exercise tolerance.
4. What is the relationship between exercise tolerance and a person's ability to participate in a regular exercise program?
5. Finish the following statement: Posture is the way you _____.

6. Explain how you can tell whether your standing posture is satisfactory.
7. Explain the initials GAS.
8. How much sleep do you need each night? Is this an adequate amount? How can you tell when you have obtained an adequate amount of sleep?
9. Test your standing posture. Have someone take your photograph. Draw a line on the photograph according to the explanation given on page 65. Is your posture what it should be?

Chapter 6

TOTAL FITNESS PROGRAMS

It is important to consult a professional physical educator because he can design a balanced total fitness program that does not overemphasize one aspect of physical development. Isometric exercises have limited benefits because their value is restricted largely to the development and maintenance of muscular strength. Calisthenic exercises and weight training exercises improve both muscular endurance and muscular strength. However, these exercises have minimal value for circulatory fitness.

Brisk walking, jogging, and running are excellent circulatory exercises, but they do little for the abdominal, back, shoulder, and arm muscles. Therefore, they should be accompanied by exercises which strengthen these regions. There are few sports in which all parts of the body are exercised equally well. People who have been inactive and have a low exercise tolerance should pace themselves carefully when participating in vigorous sports. In fact, such people may want to avoid vigorous sports until they are in condition. Conditioning requires a minimum of six weeks of warming up, calisthenics, or weight training.

Women should take special care to select exercises which provide a balanced program—one which develops muscular strength, muscular endurance, and circulatory endurance. They should emphasize exercises which strengthen abdominal and back muscles and participate in sports which improve posture and balance (tennis, volleyball, etc).

Pregnant women should consult their obstetricians about exercise programs. If such programs are not too strenuous, the doctor will approve of them. Even when doctors decide that exercise is not advisable during pregnancy, women are usually able to resume exercising very shortly after they give birth.

If a pregnant woman has been participating in a regular daily exercise program which includes activities to strengthen abdominal and back muscles, she should be able to carry her child easily, deliver easily and swiftly, and rapidly regain her figure after the delivery. Normally, such a woman should be able to continue her regular exercise program up to the sixth month of the pregnancy. During the last three months, she may engage only in a simple walking program.

CALISTHENICS

Calisthenics provide the opportunity to exercise specific groups of muscles. Figures 6.1, 6.2 and 6.3 give directions for exercises which test the strength and flexibility of the muscles in the shoulder, abdomen, and back. These exercises provide a foundation from which a calisthenic program may be devloped. You should not, however, go on to more vigorous exercises (progression) until you can complete these tests.

A great variety of calisthenic programs have been developed to exercise every group of muscles in the body. Some of these are "spot" exercises which change body contours or reduce weight in specific places. No exercise affects only one part of the body but some emphasize development on one area or one muscle group. Others are series of calisthenics which exercise the whole body.

The following are a series of exercises designed to control trouble areas in men and women who are over thirty years of age. You should begin performing these early so you can do them correctly and effortlessly when you reach the thirties.

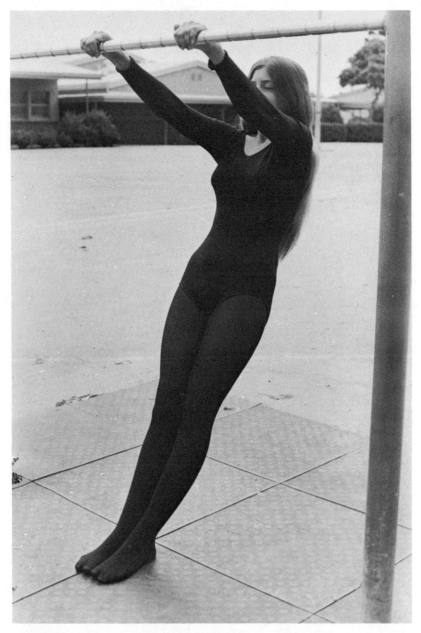

Figure 6.1 Modified pull-ups for women. *Starting position.* Grasp the bar with the palms of your hands facing outward. Extend your legs under the bar, keeping your body and knees straight. Fully extend your arms so they form an angle of 90 degrees with the body line.
Action. 1. Pull your body up until your chest touches the bar. Your body must be kept straight. 2. Lower your body until your elbows are fully extended. Your chest must touch the bar, at which time your arms must be fully extended. 3. No resting between repetitions is permitted.

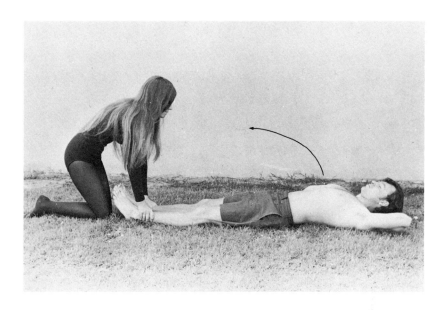

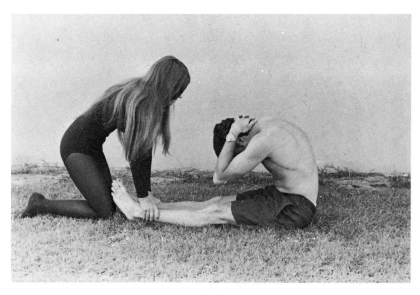

Figure 6.2 Sit-ups for men and women. *Starting position.* Lie down on your back with your legs extended, keeping your feet about 1 foot apart. Interlace your fingers and grasp the back of your neck. *Action.* 1. Sit up and turn your trunk to the left; place your right elbow on your left knee. 2. Return to the starting position. 3. Sit up and turn the trunk to the right and place your left elbow on your right knee. 4. Return to the starting position.

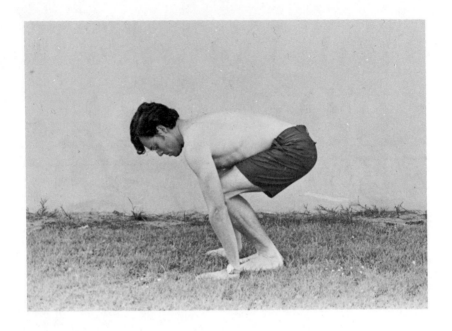

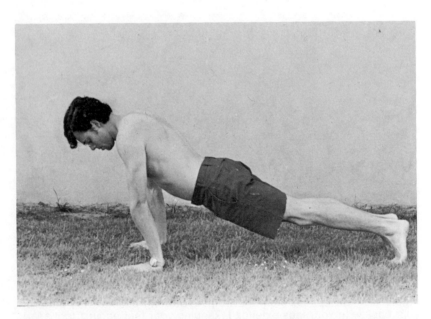

Figure 6.3 Squat thrusts for men and women. The object is to count each squat thrust for 10 seconds. *Starting position.* Stand at attention. *Action.* 1. Bend your knees and place your hands on the floor in front of your feet. 2. Thrust your legs far enough back to straighten the body from shoulders to feet (the push-up position). 3. Return to squat position. 4. Return to standing position.

Bent-knee sit-up. Do the sit-ups explained in Figure 6.4. A sit-up is one of the most important exercises an individual can perform. They reduce "spare tires" and strengthen abdominal and back muscles, thus reducing fatigue and backache. Women should start with five bent-knee sit-ups and add two a week until they are doing ten a day; men should start the same but should progress to fourteen a day. If you have trouble doing sit-ups, then do *down-rolls;* that is, reverse the procedure by starting in the sitting position, and roll down. Then get up any way you can until you build the strength to do it correctly. Do about five down-rolls a day until you can do one sit-up. Then start on the sit-up program.

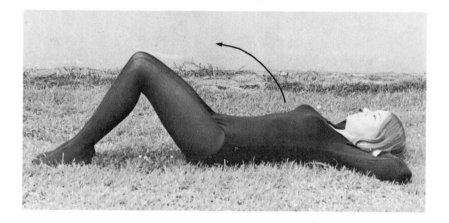

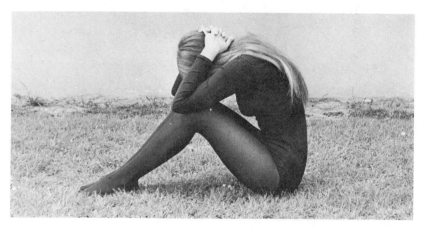

Figure 6.4 Bent-knee sit-ups. *Starting position.* Lie on your back with your hands clasped behind your head, your knees bent, and your feet held down. *Action.* 1. Keeping your chin on your chest and your back rounded, roll up into a sitting position. 2. When you are in a sitting position, straighten your back, lift your head, and press your elbows back. 3. Hold for 2 seconds, then drop your head, round your back, and roll slowly down to the starting position.

Knee-to-nose kick. This exercise, explained in Figure 6.5, is excellent for slimming the hips; it also improves the seat muscles, the lower back muscles, and the abdominal muscles. Do this exercise in sets of eight and add a set a week until the hips start to slim.

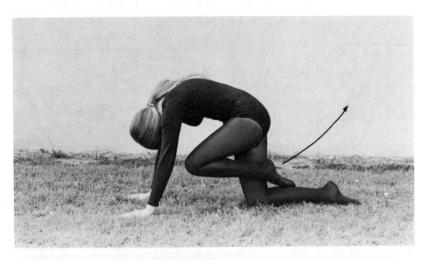

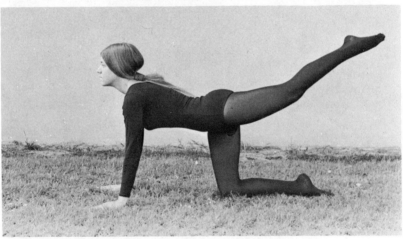

Figure 6.5 Knee-to-nose-kick. *Starting position.* Get down on your hands and knees on a soft surface. *Action.* 1. Bring your left knee as close to your nose as possible and hold it there for 2 seconds. 2. Next, extend the left leg back and up. At the same time, bring your head up. Hold for 2 seconds.

Hydrant exercise. This exercise, explained in Figure 6.6, slims the lateral sides of the hips and thighs of females. It helps to re-move fat pads which accumulate after age thirty. This is a complicated and unpleasant exercise, but it works. Do two to a side for a set. Do two sets and work up to four sets.

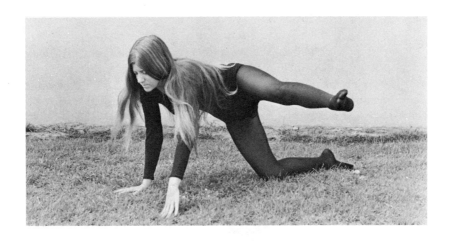

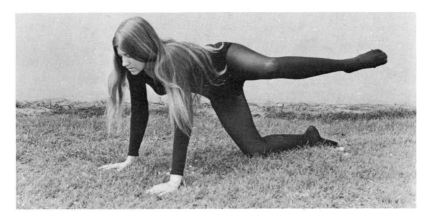

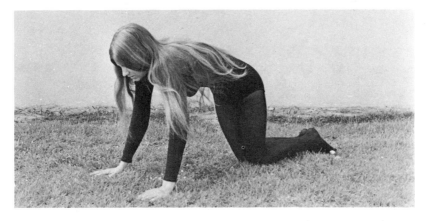

Figure 6.6 Hydrant exercise. *Starting position.* Start on your hands and knees on a soft surface. *Action. 1.* Keeping your left knee bent, raise it to the side until it is level with your hips. 2. Extend the leg straight out to the side, try to keep it at hip level. 3. Then bend the knee back and return it to the floor in the starting position.

Body rotation exercise.   These exercises trim the waist. Body rotation is explained in Figure 5.3 (page 78). To strengthen and also sharpen your neck and chinline, try to do body rotation exercises while you are standing; do not bend at the waist, and follow with your eyes the arm which is flung backward (Figure 6.7). Start with sixteen and build to thirty a day.

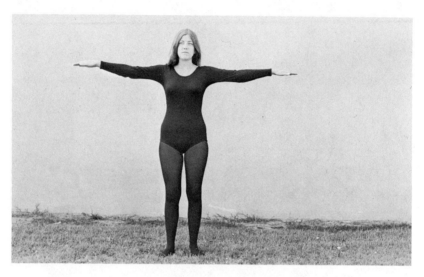

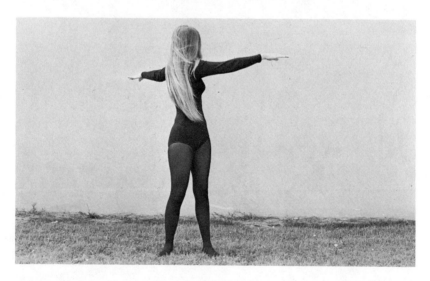

Figure 6.7 Standing body rotation. *Starting position.* Stand with your feet well apart, and extend your arms out to the sides. *Action.* 1. Twist your upper body all the way around to the right following it with your eyes; hold for 1 second. 2. Twist back to the left as far as possible; hold for 1 second.

Crossover exercises.   Crossover exercises reduce heavy thighs and increase the flexibility of the hip and ankle joints. If the thighs are very heavy and the tissue seems thick and hard, spend a minute kneading and pinching to massage them before beginning this exercise. For thighs of average size, follow the procedure explained in Figure 6.8 four times with each leg. If your thighs are heavy, start with two sets (four crossovers with each leg) and work up to as many as possible. This is the best thigh exercise there is.

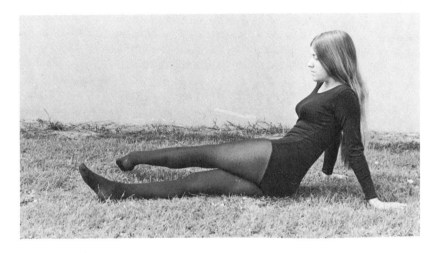

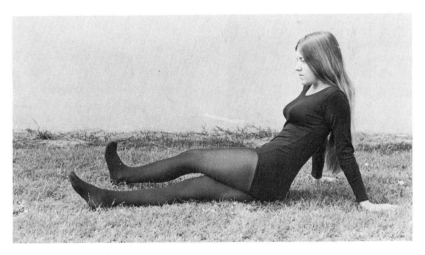

Figure 6.8   Crossover exercise. *Starting position.* Sit with legs spread apart and lean back on straightened arms. *Action.* 1. Carry the left leg across over the right leg and touch the big toe on the floor. 2. Keeping the leg in the crossed position, rotate the foot so that the toes point toward the ceiling; hold for 2 seconds. 3. Carry the left leg back over the spread-leg position and touch the floor with the little toe.

Knee bend.   Knee bends should be done by women who want to shape thin or heavy legs. If the thighs are heavy, knead and massage them for about 1 minute before beginning the exercises. Do every move explained in Figure 6.9 very slowly, to the count of four. Start with two complete knee bends and work up to fifty a day. All fifty need not be done at one time.

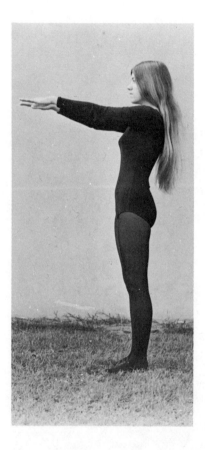 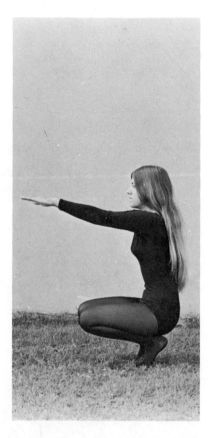

Figure 6.9   Knee bends. *Starting position.* Stand with your legs together and feet parallel. *Action.* 1. Rise to the toes for a count of 1 and bring your arms forward for balance. 2. Tighten the muscles of the seat, abdominal area, thighs, and knees. 3. Keeping your back very straight, lower yourself into a deep knee-bend. 4. Rise again to the toe position and then lower yourself to your heels.

Most people over thirty, male and female, have figure or physique problem. Pick out the problem that bot most, and work on it while doing a series of exercises for body. When the problem area is under control, pick out another one and work on it.

There are many basic calisthenic programs designed for the whole body. In the early 1960s the Royal Canadian Air Force originated two programs which have proved to be very successful. The 5BX (Five Basic Exercises) *Plan for Physical Fitness* for men and the *XBX* (a series of ten exercises) *Plan* for women are a series of relatively simple calisthenic exercises which can be done in 11 minutes each day. You should either follow an organized program like this one or have a physical educator design a program especially for you.

Whenever you exercise, begin with the warm-up exercises previously discussed. Then proceed to your basic routine, ending with special exercises for your problem areas.

WEIGHT TRAINING

Weight training does not develop circulatory endurance. It does increase muscular strength and endurance through application of the principle of *progressive resistance exercise.* In other words, as strength increases, resistance is increased. Progressive resistance occurs when a person moves a given resistance (barbells or weights) a definite number of times (repetitions).

Weight training combines weight lifting with calisthenics. Weight training programs may be as extensive or as simple as the individual desires, but they should not deviate from the principle of resistance progression. A person who simply wants to see how much he can lift may sprain muscles and joints. Weights should be increased only as strength increases. Weight training takes time; a person reaches his maximum strength only after three to five years of continuous progression.

Planning a Program

In weight training programs, repetition refers to the number of times a specific weight is to be lifted. Resistance is the amount of weight to be lifted. A set is the period during which a given number of repetitions are performed without the weights or barbells being set down.

It is impossible to select a standard starting weight which is appropriate for everyone. If you begin a weight training program, start with an amount of weight that feels comfortable when you start repetitions. If you are going to work out three times a week, you should increase the original weight by 5 or 10 pounds each week. Use the same weight for at least one week or for three workouts. Often, individuals starting their second workouts find themselves stiff, sore, and tired, and the weights feel heavier than they did during the first workout. If this happens to you, reduce the weights by 5 pounds for one week or by 10 pounds for two weeks; continue the reduction until the weights feel comfortable. Then progress to the point at which you began, and continue on ahead, gradually increasing the weights. This principle should also be used when you return to your weight training program after a short layoff.

Work out three times a week on alternate days, giving yourself a two-day rest at the end of the week. You may, for example, work out on Monday, Wednesday, and Friday or on Tuesday, Thursday, and Saturday. An exercise session should last from one and a half to two hours. You should perform about eight or ten different exercises and three sets of each exercise. Rest about 1 minute between sets and approximately 2 to 3 minutes between exercises. At each set increase the weight you are lifting by 5 to 10 pounds.

Plan your program in writing. Make out a program card on which you list your exercises, your starting poundage, the number of repetitions, and the number of sets. As you increase the weights in each exercise, mark the changes on your card. The program card may be referred to before and during the workout. You may also use it to make changes in your program.

Every month or six weeks, change your exercises. Substitute different exercises for the ones you have been doing until you have done all the exercises in your program. Then return to the ones you started with. Such program changes help you to maintain your interest, and they vary the pressure and resistance on each muscle.

A Weight Training Program

If you are interested in weight training, you may want to follow the trial program presented in this section. You should remain in it for three months to determine whether there is an improvement in strength. Work out three times a week on alternate days. Start with a weight (Table 6.1) which is light enough for you to do ten repetitions comfortably. Perform the exercises in their numbered order, doing one set of each. Increase the poundage whenever the weight in any one exercise feels light. Always perform the exercises in their numbered order, and do only one set of ten repetitions at each workout. While following this program, do not engage in any other regularly scheduled exercise program.

The exercises in our program are listed below (refer to Table 6.1 for recommended weights):

1. *Two arm standing press.* Stand with weight at your shoulder. Now, using the strength of the arm, shoulder, and upper back only, push the weight above your head. Lower to your shoulder and repeat. one set, 10 reps, 30 lbs

Table 6.1 Suggested Poundages at the Beginning of Weight Training

EXERCISE	AVERAGE POUNDS TO START WITH	RANGE OF CHOICE OF STARTING WEIGHT
Two arm standing press	40	30-50
Rowing motion	35	25-45
Shrug	45	35-60
Squat	45	35-55
Rise on toes	45	35-60
Lateral bench raise	7½ each	5-10 each
Barbell curl	35	25-45
Lateral raise (standing)	7½ each	5-10 each
Side bending	35	30-40
Two arm press	45	35-60
Stiff-legged dead lift	55	45-70
One arm pullover	7½ each	5-10
One arm swing	30	20-40
One arm rowing motion	20	12-15
Wrist curl	25	20-30
Reverse wrist curl	15	10-20
Thumb front wrist curl	15	10-20
Double wrist curl with straight arm	35	25-45
Two arm reverse wrist curl	25	20-35
Forward raise (standing)	15	10-20
Backward raise (body bend forward)	7½ each	5-10 each
Lateral raise (body bend forward)	7½ each	5-10 each
Straight arm pullover	7½ each	5-10 each
Pull-up to waist	35	25-45
Two arm press lying down	60	45-70
Half squat	25	20-30

2. *Rowing motion.* Stand with your legs apart and your body in front bending position; keep your arms straight down. Without any body motion, pull the weights up until the bar touches your chest. Lower and repeat.

3. *Shrug.* Hold weight while standing with arms straight out. Keeping your elbows straight, pull your shoulders up towards your ears; do not move your whole body. Relax and repeat.

4. *Squat.* Stand erect with weight held across your shoulder. Keeping your heels on floor, bend your knees until your thighs are parallel to the floor. Keep your back as straight as possible. Rise to the standing position and repeat.

5. *Rise on toes.* After performing the squat, do not remove the weight from your shoulders. Rise up on your toes and lower your heels back to the ground. Repeat.

6. *Lateral bench raise.* Lie on your back on a bench. Start with a pair of dumbbells held straight up at arm's length. Breathe in deeply, and slowly lower the weights to your side. Return to starting position and repeat.

7. *Barbell curl.* Hold weight at your thighs with both your hands. Without moving your body motion except to bend your elbows, raise the weight to the shoulders. Lower and repeat.

8. *Standing Lateral Raise.* Hold a pair of dumbbells down the sides at arms length. Keeping your elbows stiff, raise the dumbbells straight out from your shoulders. Bring the pairs together above your head. Lower and repeat.

9. *Neck exercise.* Take a light dumbbell and wrap a towel around the handle. Place it on your forehead, and raise and lower your head up and down.

10. *Side Bend.* Hold a weight in one hand and place the other hand behind your head. As you hold the weight, bend as far as you can to the side. Return to a standing position and repeat. Do this exercise for both sides.

11. *Sit-up.* Lie on the ground and hook your feet under a barbell. Raise your body to a sitting position. Lower and repeat.

Remember that hard work is required to obtain results and results occur very slowly. The trial program outlined here should begin to increase your strength within three to six months. If you enjoy this program, ask a physical educator to design a weight training program for you from one of the following tables. Such programs are often part of a college or university curriculum, a men's club, the YMCA, or a gym.

Program 1: Weight Training Exercises

EXERCISE	ACTION AND MUSCLE GROUP
1. Two arm curl 30 lbs	For the biceps of the upper arm
2. Two arm press 30	For the triceps and deltoids
3. Rowing motion 25	For the latissimus dorsi
4. Deep knee bend	For the front thigh muscles
5. Lateral raise (lying)	For the major pectorals
6. Stiff-legged dead lift	For the spinal erectors and rear thigh muscles
7. Rising on toes	For the gastrocnemius and soleus
8. Sit-up	For the straight abdominals
9. Lateral raise (standing) 5	For the deltoids
10. Side bending 30 (each side)	For the external oblique abdominals and the spinal erectors
11. One arm pullover	For the major pectoral and latissimus dorsi
12. Neck bridging	For the rear neck muscles
13. Shoulder shrug 30	For the trapezius
14. Resistance head movement	For the front neck muscles
15. Reverse wrist curl	For the extensor forearm muscles

Program 2: Weight Training Exercises

EXERCISE	ACTION AND MUSCLE GROUP
1. Thumb front curl	For the biceps and brachioradialis
2. Backward raise with body bent forward	For the rear deltoid, triceps, and latissimus dorsi
3. Lateral raise with body bent forward	For the deltoids and upper back muscles
4. One leg half-squat	For the glutius maximus and upper thigh muscles
5. Two arm press in supine position	For the major pectorals and triceps
6. Rising on toes	For the gastrocnemius and soleus
7. Sit-up	For the straight abdominals
8. Forward raise standing	For the front deltoids
9. Side bending	For the external oblique abdominals and the spinal erectors
10. One arm pullover	For the major pectoral and latissimus dorsi
11.. Resistance head movement	For the rear neck muscles
12. Shoulder shrug	For the trapezius
13. Resistance head movement	For the front neck muscles
14. Double wrist curl with straight arms	For the flexor and extensor forearm muscles

Program 3: Weight Training Exercises

EXERCISE	ACTION AND MUSCLE GROUP
1. Two arm reverse curl	For the biceps and forearm extensors
2. Two arm press from behind neck	For the triceps
3. One arm rowing motion	For the latissimus dorsi
4. Squat	For the front thigh muscles
5. Lateral raise (lying)	For the major pectorals
6. One arm swing	For the spinal erectors
7. Rising on toes	For the gastrocnimius and soleus
8. Sit-up	For the straight abdominals
9. Side bending	For the external oblique abdominals and the spinal erectors
10. Pull-up to waist	For the latissimus dorsi
11. Neck bridging	For the rear neck muscles
12. Shoulder shrug	For the trapezius
13. Resistance head movement	For the front neck muscles
14. Wrist curl	For the flexor forearm muscles

EXERCISES FOR CIRCULATORY ENDURANCE

As you have learned, circulatory endurance, or stamina, is the ability of the body to perform under stress without undue fatigue.

Circulatory endurance is attained through physical activity in which the circulatory and respiratory systems are stimulated for relatively long periods of time. The normal, healthy heart cannot be injured by such exercise and will respond beneficially to the demands placed on it. However, individuals engaging in a planned circulatory endurance program should progress in graduated increments and should avoid placing drastic demands on their hearts. An individual may determine whether or not he is exercising safely by taking his pulse rate periodically during endurance exercises. The pulse rate should never rise above 151 beats per minute for people under thirty years of age or above 131 beats per minute for people over thirty. If individuals will engage in activities which increase their pulse rates to these maximums and if they sustain such activities for 15 minutes four times a week, they will improve their circulatory endurance to an adequate level.

Walking, Jogging, and Running

Each year many deaths from cardiac failure occur because of jogging and running. These deaths occur because people with heart defects placed excessive demands on their hearts. Anyone with a known or suspected heart or lung disability should exercise only under the direction of a physician. All apparently well individuals over thirty years of age should be considered as having a suspected heart or lung disability until a physician has proven otherwise. Graduated increments of walking, jogging, and running, done after a physical examination and with medical approval, improve appearance and endurance. Such a program can provide energy for the enjoyment of life and help to prevent fatigue.

Walking is the most natural of all forms of exercise. A person may walk at any time with almost no medical risk. Brisk walking accelerates the pulse and strengthens the heart, lungs, and legs. Extremely inactive people may obtain some endurance effects by walking; later, however, they must increase their rate of speed to obtain further benefits. Inactive, sedentary men (more than women) over fifty years of age should walk for exercise; they should not try jogging or running because of the increased chance of heart attack after fifty.

Jogging, the next step up from walking, is steady, slow running. Jogging may be alternated with breath-catching periods of walking. Jogging became popular in the late 1960s with the publication of *Jogging* by William J. Bowerman, track coach at the University of Oregon, and W. E. Harris, M.D., a heart specialist. This book presents a detailed, complete program for anyone interested in jogging as part of his exercise program. Jogging is pleasant, free, easy, relaxing, and fun. It can be done alone or in groups. Jogging is especially good for maintaining circulatory endurance. To achieve this purpose, however, it must be alternated with intervals of hard running after the first month or two of progression.

A jogging program begins with a short period of trotting and walking. As jogging progresses, the jogger covers greater and greater distances. You may want to attempt the following trial program for one month. If you enjoy it, obtain the book *Jogging* or ask a physical educator to design a program for you.

Schedule I Week 1 (Total Distance: ½ Mile)

Monday	Warm up (always do warm-up exercises). Jog 55 yards in 25-30 seconds; then walk 55 yards.[a] Repeat four times.
Tuesday	Walk for 5-10 minutes after warming up.
Wednesday	Jog 110 yards in 55-60 seconds; then walk 110 yards.
Thursday	Walk for 5-10 minutes after warming up.
Friday	Jog 55 yards in 25-30 seconds; then walk 55 yards. Repeat two times.
Saturday and Sunday	Walk for 5-10 minutes after warming up.

Schedule I Week 2 (Total Distance: ¾ Mile)

Monday	Jog 55 yards in 25-30 seconds; then walk 55 yards. Repeat four times.
	Jog 110 yards in 55-60 seconds; then walk 110 yards. Repeat four times.
	Jog 55 yards in 25-30 seconds; then walk 55 yards. Repeat four times.
Wednesday	Jog 55 yards in 25-30 seconds; then walk 55 yards. Repeat three times.
	Jog 110 yards in 55-60 seconds; then walk 110 yards. Repeat three times.
	Jog 55 yards in 25-30 seconds; then walk 55 yards. Repeat three times.
Friday	Jog 55 yards in 25-30 seconds; then walk 55 yards. Repeat four times.
	Jog 110 yards in 55-60 seconds; then walk 110 yards. Repeat two times.
	Jog 55 yards in 25-30 seconds; then walk 55 yards. Repeat four times.

[a]You need only estimate distances; they do not have to be accurate. A track is usually 440 yards in length with each straightaway and turn 110 yards. Using a car odometer or a pedometer, lay out a course beforehand. City blocks are about 220 feet by 500 feet. Telephone poles are about 100 yards apart. Any watch with a second hand is adequate for timing.

Schedule II   Week 2 (Total Distance: 1 Mile)

Monday	Jog 55 yards in 25-30 seconds; then walk 55 yards. Repeat four times.
	Jog 110 yards in 55-60 seconds; then walk 110 yards. Repeat four times.
	Jog 55 yards in 25-30 seconds; then walk 55 yards. Repeat four times.
Wednesday	Jog 55 yards in 25-30 seconds; then walk 55 yards. Repeat three times.
	Jog 110 yards in 55-60 seconds; then walk 110 yards. Repeat five times.
	Jog 55 yards in 25-30 seconds; then walk 55 yards. Repeat three times.
Friday	Jog 55 yards in 25-30 seconds; then walk 55 yards. Repeat two times.
	Jog 110 yards in 55-60 seconds; then walk 110 yards. Repeat six times.
	Jog 55 yards in 25-30 seconds; then walk 55 yards. Repeat four times.

Schedule I   Week 3 (Total Distance: 1 Mile)

Monday	Jog 55 yards in 22-25 seconds, then walk 55 yards. Repeat four times.
	Jog 220 yards in 90-100 seconds, then walk 220 yards. Repeat one time.
	Jog 110 yards in 45-50 seconds, then walk 110 yards. Repeat two times.
	Jog 55 yards in 22-25 seconds, then walk 55 yards. Repeat four times.
Wednesday	Jog 55 yards in 22-25 seconds, then walk 55 yards. Repeat two times.
	Start a slow, steady jog for 2 or 3 minutes. The pace is 55 to 75 seconds for 110 yards. Walk whenever you need to; walk at the end of the 3 minutes. Jog again steadily for 2 or 3 minutes. Jog 55 yards in 22-25 seconds, then walk 55 yards. Repeat two times.
Friday	Jog 55 yards in 22-55 seconds, then walk 55 yards. Repeat two times.
	Jog 110 yards in 45-50 seconds, then walk 110 yards. Repeat one time.
	Jog your slow, steady pace for 2 or 3 minutes. Then walk until wind is back to normal.
	Jog 55 yards in 22-25 seconds, then walk 55 yards. Repeat two times.

Schedules are planned for Monday, Wednesday, and Friday. You may rearrange them (Tuesday, Thursday, and Saturday) to fit your own schedule if you will remember the "hard-easy" principle of all exercise programs—exercise one day, rest the next. No exercise program should be followed every day. If you jog for 55 yards and it leaves you gasping and too breathless to talk with your fellow joggers, you are running too fast or you have not worked yourself into the condition to perform in this program. (For conditioning exercises, turn to page 76.) If the 110-yard jogs were not too much for you, try Schedule II in the second week. If the first week's schedule seemed comfortable and you were pleased with your performance, continue on Schedule I for the second week.

Schedule II   Week 3 (Total Distance: 1¼ Miles)

Monday	Jog 55 yards in 22-30 seconds, then walk 55 yards. Repeat four times.
	Jog 110 yards in 45-60 seconds, then walk 110 yards. Repeat two times.
	Jog 220 yards in 90-100 seconds, then walk 220 yards. Repeat two times.
	Jog 110 yards in 45-60 seconds, then walk 110 yards. Repeat two times.
Wednesday	Start to establish a steady, comfortable jogging pace for the required distance. Start at about 110 yards in 56 seconds. This is 4 miles per hour. See how long you can continuously jog with comfort. Walk when too winded to talk with companions. Jog and walk for 1¼ miles.
Friday	Jog 110 yards in 45-50 seconds, then walk 110 yards. Repeat four times.
	Jog steadily 330 yards in 2 minutes 48 seconds. Walk until wind is back to normal.
	Jog 110 yards in 45-50 seconds, then walk 110 yards. Repeat four times.

By the fourth week you should know whether jogging is an exercise program that you enjoy. Also, you will know enough about it to use it for change of pace in other exercise programs. Exercise must be fun if an individual is to continue on with it. Therefore, expose yourself to a number of different exercise programs. You may maintain your interest in fitness activities by alternating exercises if one set of exercises begins to bore you.

Schedule I   Week 4 (Total Distance: 1 Mile)

At this point you may want to begin jogging steadily. Jog for 2-3 minutes. Walk until wind is back to normal. Repeat for 1 mile.

Schedule II   Week 4 (Total Distance: 1½ Miles)

Slow, comfortable, steady jogging. Walk whenever you are too winded to talk to companions. Walk until wind is back to normal. Repeat cycles until you have jogged 1½ miles.

If you decide to continue jogging, refer to William J. Bowerman's book *Jogging*. It provides schedules for reaching 4 or 5 miles a day. It also contains complete programs and many suggestions for varying your program to maintain interest.

Jogging may be satisfactory to an individual during the initial phase of conditioning. After the goal of 1 mile is achieved, however, running often replaces jogging. Running can provide a challenge as well as good circulatory endurance. The progression of jogging and walking outlined previously may be used to progress toward the goal of running 1 mile. Some people, however, may want to increase the time period in the schedule to two months. Before you try to run a mile, be sure that you can jog comfortably for this distance. Don't worry about your time at first. When you can jog for a mile, start pacing yourself and reducing your time. You should pace yourself so that you are running at a constant rate. Avoid any bursts of speed because they greatly reduce your efficiency and cause fatigue. Reduce your time by 10 seconds a week until you can run a mile in 6 minutes. This is considered excellent time for maintenance of circulatory endurance.

When space or weather restricts your ability to run, running in place can be a very effective means of maintaining circulatory endurance. The important factors in running in place are the cadence of the step and the duration of the activity. The most comfortable time length seems to be 5 minutes. To reach a 5-minute goal, begin by running in place for 1 minute. Then increase your time by 30-second intervals. Run for five sessions at each time level before progressing to the next interval.

NUMBER OF SESSIONS	RUNNING TIME
1-5	1 minute
6-10	1½ minutes
11-15	2 minutes
16-20	2½ minutes
21-25	3 minutes
26-30	3½ minutes
31-35	4 minutes
36-40	4½ minutes
41-45	5 minutes

When you can run in place for 5 minutes, you may begin to increase your step cadence.

Aerobics

Aerobics is a total fitness program first published in 1968. The originator of the program was Major Kenneth H. Cooper, M.D., of the U. S. Air Force Medical Corps. The key concept in this program is oxygen consumption. Because oxygen cannot be stored in the body, it must be continually replenished (Chapter 1). Consequently, the fatigue level of an individual is controlled by the ability of his respiratory and circulatory systems to supply oxygen to the muscles.

Distances Covered in 12 Minutes by Running

AGE GROUPS	FITNESS CATEGORIES	AGE GROUPS
Under 30 years		30 to 39 years
Less than 1.0 mile	Very poor	Less than 0.95 mile
1.0 to 1.24 miles	Poor	0.95 to 1.14 miles
1.25 to 1.49 miles	Fair	1.15 to 1.39 miles
1.50 to 1.74 miles	Good	1.40 to 1.64 miles
1.75 miles and over	Excellent	1.65 miles and over
40 to 49 years		Over 50 years
Less than 0.85 mile	Very poor	Less than 0.80 mile
0.85 to 1.04 miles	Poor	0.80 to 0.99 miles
1.05 to 1.29 miles	Fair	1.00 to 1.24 miles
1.30 to 1.54 miles	Good	1.25 to 1.49 miles
1.55 miles and over	Excellent	1.50 miles and over

Dr. Cooper's aerobics system consists of a point count assigned to different physical activities that increase circulatory endurance. In his physical activities an individual progresses to the point where he can perform activities worth thirty points each week. The number of points represents the amount of the physical activity necessary for maintenance of the cardiorespiratory system.

Points are obtained by performing specific circulatory endurance activities in a specific amount of time. Such activities include running, swimming, bicycling, walking, running in place, and participating in strenuous games of squash, handball, and basketball. Dr. Cooper's book *The New Aerobics* (a revised version of the program published in 1968) provides standards against which a person may gauge his aerobic fitness. For beginners to the program the test of aerobic fitness is the distance that can be covered by running in 12 minutes.

After you have determined your fitness category, refer to *The New Aerobics* and choose the schedule you should follow to obtain thirty aerobic points per week.

CIRCUIT TRAINING

Circuit refers to a number of carefully selected exercises which are arranged and numbered consecutively; the exercises range over a given area. Each numbered exercise within the circuit is called a *station*. An individual moves at his own speed from one station to another until he completes the entire circuit. In most cases he repeats the total circuit more than once (usually three times) and records the total time of performance. This is a convenient and different approach to exercising—one that is physically, physiologically, and psychologically sound.

Circuit training involves two valuable activities. The best physical activity for development of muscular strength and muscular endurance is weight training. The most effective methods for developing and maintaining circulatory and respiratory endurance involve running (exceptions are swimming, bicycling, and rope skipping). Some people are able to participate quite regularly in either weight training or running, but very seldom are they able to participate in both. A well-planned circuit involves both weight training and running. Thus circuit training increases muscular strength, muscular endurance, and cardiovascular endurance.

In circuit training elaborate or expensive equipment is not always necessary. In many circuits almost no equipment is used. At the other extreme are those circuits made up entirely of exercises requiring special equipment such as barbells, dumbbells, ladders, and gymnastic apparatus. The most common circuits are a combination of these two extremes, with some stations requiring equipment and others requiring none.

The value of circuit training lies in its extreme adaptability to a great variety of situations. A circuit can be designed to fit any individual, group, area, or condition (it is even adaptable to medical rehabilitation). Circuit training enables an individual or a group of people to progress through a series of exercises and check the progress against a clock.

When circuit training is used in schools, the student knows in advance exactly what he will be required to do. Furthermore, circuits may be tailored to fit each individual in the class. Consequently, students can work alone or in groups without direction from the instructor. During classroom instruction an individual should be taught how to plan and construct his own circuit for use outside of class.

Circuit training utilizes three variables: load, repetitions, and time. Weight training exercises provide the load, and sets provide the repetitions. Interval running, engaged in between stations, provides repetitions and time.

On a circuit, progression is produced by decreasing the time required to complete one circuit, increasing the work load (weight or sets), or a combination of both. Progression is assured because an individual works at his present capacity and can progress as his capacity increases. Circuit training provides a series of progressive time goals which are achieved step by step. This time factor provides built-in motivation; it encourages a person to push himself to do better. The circuit layout in which a person moves from one station to another offers variety; this is appealing to most people.

The progressions used in weight training may be used in circuit training if loads can be increased by progressively increasing the size of the weights to be lifted. In circuit training it is not necessary to change weights as frequently as it is in weight training because weight training is only one of the variables involved in the program.

Calisthenic exercises may be used in a circuit. When this is done, the load is a person's own body weight. The load is increased by modifying the exercise. For example, the following changes will increase the work load in a push-up: standard push-up; push-up, pushing hands off the floor; push-up, pushing off the floor and clapping hands; pushing up, pushing off the floor and slapping the chest. Such modifications make calisthenic exercises very useful in circuit training. Load can also be increased by increasing the number of repetitions, or sets, at each station or by increasing the number of times the circuit is run. Laps may be added; in that case, a person runs the length of the circuit without performing at the stations. Another way to increase the load is to decrease the time needed to perform a circuit. In maintaining good progression the most important factor is to increase the work load gradually and at a rate that can be handled with ease and safety.

Planning a Circuit

An individual should know his goals before beginning any exercise program. He should be able to say what purpose he wants the program to serve. In planning a circuit, remember that your circuit must be based on your personal goals.

In planning a circuit, choose exercises that are strenuous. Each exercise should contribute toward progression by increasing both work load and work rate. This automatically eliminates the very light warm-up exercises which should be performed before the circuit is run. Do not include "duck waddle," deep knee bends, or any other exercise which can cause joint, ligament, or muscle damage if done too fast.

Standardize the exercises so that you know how much work you are doing and are able to observe and evaluate your improvement. Also, perform each exercise the same way every time.

Select exercises that balance other exercises so that all groups of muscles receive proper exercise. Improper balance of strength between antagonistic muscle groups can produce permanent body damage. To avoid improper balance, classify the muscle groups into three categories: the arm, neck, and shoulder group; the abdomen, back and chest group; and the buttock, hip, and leg group. When arranging your stations, avoid consecutive placement of exercises that involve similar muscle groups. For example, both arm curls and chin-ups involve the arm, neck, and shoulder muscle group. If you include both these exercises in a circuit, separate them. A circuit designed for general body conditioning should include exercises which involve all three of the muscle groups.

Although you perform against time, do not rush around the circuit at such a reckless pace that it becomes a race against the clock. Exercises may be harmful and ineffective if they are performed incorrectly.

The amount of time you have available for performing a circuit is a factor in determining both the difficulty of exercises and the number of stations to be included in the circuit. The spacing and the arrangement of the stations are determined by the amount of space you have available and by the kinds of exercises you want to emphasize. If your basic purpose is general body conditioning (an emphasis on cardiovascular endurance), you should choose a large area for your circuit, allowing for distances between stations for running and movement. There should always be enough room for exercise which is strenuous, yet free-flowing and uninterrupted. Where there is available space and facilities, several circuits (or variations of one circuit) may be organized, utilizing the same area or equipment.

The following patterns are examples of circuits useful for general body conditioning. However, a person with a little experience, skill, and understanding may design circuits to meet the fitness needs of nearly any vigorous sport or activity.

The circuit in Table 6.2 provides for progression through increased repetitions. In the circuit in Table 6.3 no equipment is used, and progression can be produced by increasing repetitions or decreasing circuit time. The following is a short 10-minute circuit which utilizes some of the exercises discussed in this chapter. Follow the recommendations listed at each exercise for progression. Determine your own time limit by judging how well you perform the circuit when you first try it.

1. Squat (page 97)
2. Barbell curl (page 98)
3. Sit-ups (Figure 6.4)
4. Knee bends (Figure 6.9)
5. Wrist curl (Table 6.1)
6. Knee-to-nose kick (Figure 6.5)
7. Straight arm pullover (Table 6.1)
8. Step-ups onto chairs or benches (with weights)

These are merely examples; any number of exercises can be used. See how skillful you can be in designing your own exercises for your circuit.

Table 6.2 Recommended Circuit

EXERCISES		REPETITIONS			
ORDER	KIND	1	2	3	WEIGHT IN POUNDS
1.	Bench press	8	10	12	60
2.	Side bends	7	9	11	
3.	Chins	1	3	5	
4.	Back extension	7	9	12	10
5.	Two arm curl	8	10	12	25
6.	Squat	10	13	16	
7.	Bent leg sit-ups	15	20	25	
8.	Three-quarter squat	9	12	15	25
9.	Lateral raise	8	10	12	7½
10.	Shuttle run	(5-10 yards)			

Table 6.3 Circuit Training Pattern Using No Apparatus

1. Step-ups (use chairs, benches, or bleachers) — *one minute each station*
2. Isometric arm exercises[a] — *in btw running on*
3. Squat thrusts *the spot 1 min*
4. ~~Body rotations~~
5. Isometric back exercises[a] *jumping jacks*
6. Push-ups *rising on toes*
7. Bent-knee sit-ups *rope skipping*
8. ~~Shuttle run (5-10 yards)~~

[a]There are so many isometric exercises that you may devise one for this specific area.

ROPE SKIPPING

Rope skipping is an excellent cardiovascular exercise. A person who jumps steadily for 5 minutes is getting a good workout. A 10-minute daily program of rope skipping improves and maintains cardiovascular endurance as well as a 30-minute program of jogging. Rope skipping may be either a program in itself or a bad-weather substitute for a jogging, running program.

Rope is inexpensive. Cut a piece which is anywhere from 6 to 9 feet long; the correct length is the one most comfortable for you. Tape the ends so they will not fray.

Variations within a rope skipping program can add interest and incentive. They may also provide progression. (Progression may also be achieved by performing a specific number of jumps in a certain amount of time.) The normal skipping style may be modified by jumping on one foot, alternating feet, or jumping with both feet together. Running while skipping increases timing and coordination. Jumping backward is a simple maneuver in which various foot styles can be used. Make some forward-to-backward changes and then some backward-to-forward changes. This is difficult because you must jump an extra time as the turn is completed.

A double jump is challenging. This is done by spinning the rope faster and jumping a little higher. When you have increased your skill, shorten the rope slightly by winding it within the hand, and stay in the air longer by bending the knees and keeping them high. You may achieve a triple jump. Double and triple jumps have an effect similar to that caused by sprints in running; they rapidly increase the heart rate.

A front cross may be achieved by crossing the arms when the rope starts downward. This makes a loop through which you may jump. On completion of the jump, the arms are uncrossed and the next jump is made in the normal manner. If you have difficulty performing a front cross, lengthen the rope slightly and either lower the hands as the arms cross or cross the arms far enough to bring the elbows together. These changes will give you a wider loop to jump through. A back cross may be done by performing a regular back jump with arms crossed in front of the body (cross your arms so your elbows touch each other).

Make your own modifications. Try jumps such as a double jump with a front cross, or try to run while you change jumping forms. Again, make some forward-to-backward changes and then some backward-to-forward changes.

SPORTS

Sports and other recreational activities may serve as conditioning programs. However, some individual and dual sports require such small amounts of physical activity that they are not adequate for a fitness program. Golf is such a sport. It has many psychological and social values but little physical value. The main energy expenditure in golf comes from walking. This walking is usually not vigorous enough to elevate the pulse significantly.

If a sport is to supply the requirements of a physical fitness program, it must be vigorous. Also, a person should participate in it for at least three sessions a week. Each session should last for a minimum of 30 minutes. Ideally, a person who is using a sport as the basis of a fitness program should participate in the sport for 60 minutes every day.

When you participate in a sport, you should remember that your expenditure of energy depends on several factors:

1. *The number of participants.* In calisthenics, weight training, and running, you control the expenditure of energy. In dual sports,

however, you must consider the number of participants. Ha1
be least demanding in a game of doubles, more demanding
of singles, and most demanding in a game involving th
("cutthroat").

2. *The skill of the participants.* Generally, a high level of skill
is reflected in greater efficiency. Thus a skilled person can participate
at a lower energy cost. As your skill develops, you should either increase the amount of time you devote to a sport or pit yourself against
people who are more skillful than you are.

3. *The duration.* The longer the duration of an activity, the
greater is the energy expenditure. Each participant should be vigorously active for 30 to 40 minutes; in a 60-minute game, then, you
should be moving one-half to two-thirds of the time.

4. *The speed of the necessary physical movements.* Sports
which require occasional bursts of speed are more demanding and require a greater expenditure of energy then are sports in which the participants can establish a steady pace. You should participate in such
sports only after you feel your physical condition is adequate.

In choosing sports, remember the value of developing and
maintaining circulatory endurance. Sports which improve circulatory
endurance include individual activities such as swimming, scuba div-
ing, snorkeling, hiking, running, and bicycling; dual activities such as
wrestling, and judo; and court games such as badminton, handball,
squash, tennis, and volleyball.

Dual sports and court games require at least two participants.
Court games further require a court. These requirements may limit
your opportunities to engage in exercise. Individual activities usually
offer more opportunities for participation.

Some sports are much more beneficial to fitness than are
others. Golf is the least beneficial. It is followed, in increasing benefit,
by court games, dual sports, individual sports, weight training, jogging,
and running.

USE OF LEISURE TIME

Today, most leisure hours are spent in front of a television
set. Time spent in this way is not physically or psychologically beneficial. Physical activities have psychological, as well as physiological,
benefits. Exercise helps you to feel good, act decisively, and retain a
positive and confident outlook on life. Participation in activities which
give you an opportunity to be a part of nature is both enjoyable and
healthy. Begin to spend your leisure time in activities that will help to
reacquaint you with the environment.

1. *Spend time in your garden.* Feel the pride which comes

from growing beautiful flowers or your own vegetables. Learn how our ecological system operates.

2. *Discover the pleasure of walking.* Take time to see the many sights in your neighborhood. Discover parks, mountains, and seashores, and learn to appreciate nature.

3. *Take up hiking.* Take small walking trips in the hills, maybe with a picnic lunch. If hiking in earnest appeals to you, seek out the nearest chapter of the Sierra Club, Appalachian Club, or some other nature organization. Such clubs provide information about hiking and hiking equipment.

4. *Go camping.* Try it with the bare essentials. Do not try backpacking (carrying everything you need in a pack on your back) without seeking professional guidance. This can be very dangerous. Here, again, the Sierra Club has training programs for backpacking.

5. *Start to bicycle.* Short rides out from your home will show you areas that you did not know existed. Obtain a bicycle carrier for your car. Then you can drive to places of interest and use the bicycle for touring. From a bicycle, countryside seems much different than it does from a car.

6. *If you purchase a boat, buy a canoe, kayak, or sailboat instead of a motorboat.* They do not contribute to pollution and they provide you with an opportunity for physical activity.

7. *Participate in winter sports instead of spending the winter in front of a television set.* Jogging and running require continuous expenditures of large amounts of energy and, thus, may lead to exhaustion in a short period of time. Downhill skiing involves lower energy expenditures (25 to 40 per cent maximum), and it provides frequent interruptions and rests and time to view the scenery. Trade off your snowmobile for some snowshoes or crosscountry skis, and do some winter touring.

All of these activities provide healthy exercise, bring you close to your natural environment, are pleasurable, and cost much less than motor-driven recreational vehicles.

Take an active interest in biology, ecology, and geology. Knowledge in these fields will help you become aware of your surroundings and will greatly enhance your appreciation of nature. The natural environment is fragile, yet resilient. It is easy to upset its delicate balance, but it will withstand abuse for a long period of time before it is destroyed. If natural areas are treated with respect, they will remain in good condition, and large numbers of people can visit and enjoy them.

Machines such as trail bikes, motorboats, snowmobiles, and jeeps often abuse the environment. They cause pollution and may destroy plants.

Don't litter. Everything carried into an area should be carried back out. There should be no such thing as garbage in a natural area.

When camping, carry your own stove and fuel. Mountain areas are now so heavily used that there is no longer enough dead wood to enable you to forage for fuel.

All people should have the chance to see the natural world and to understand the natural support system that sustains life. Cleaning up a lake, a stream, or a beach area makes sense to someone who spent time in a wilderness area. Only after people have spent time in natural surroundings will they understand the importance of conservation. Then they may find ways to bring their life styles back into harmony with the natural environment.

SUMMARY

I. It is important to consult a physical educator because he can design a balanced program that does not overemphasize one aspect of physical development.
   A. Women should take special care to select exercises which provide a balanced program.
   B. Exercise During Pregnancy
      1. A woman should consult her obstetrician about an exercise program during pregnancy.
      2. Most women should be able to continue their regular exercise programs up to the sixth month of pregnancy.
II. Calisthenic Exercises
   A. The value of calisthenics is that you can exercise specific groups of muscles.
   B. Calisthenic Programs. A great variety of calisthenic programs have been developed to exercise every group of muscles on the body.
      1. The following are a series of exercises designed to control trouble areas in men and women:
         a. Bent-knee sit-up.
         b. Knee-to-knee kicks.
         c. Hydrant exercise.
         d. Body rotation exercise.
         e. Crossover exercise.
         f. Knee bends.
      2. The Royal Canadian Air Force exercises are successful for men and women.
III. Weight Training (a combination of weight lifting and calisthenics)
   A. Planning a Program

1. It is impossible to select a standard starting weight which is appropriate for everyone. Begin with the amount of weight that feels comfortable to you.
2. Work out three times a week on alternate days.
3. Plan your program in writing; make out a program card.

B. The following is a trial weight training program. You should remain in it for three months to determine whether there are improvements in strength.
   1. Two arm standing press
   2. Rowing motion
   3. Shrug
   4. Squat
   5. Rise on toes
   6. Lateral bench raise
   7. Barbell curl
   8. Standing lateral raise
   9. Neck exercise
   10. Side bend
   11. Sit-up

IV. Exercises for Circulatory Endurance

A. Walking, jogging, and running, done in graduated increments, may improve appearance and endurance. Such a program may provide energy for the enjoyment of life and help to prevent fatigue.
   1. Walking is the most natural of all forms of exercise.
   2. Jogging is a steady, easy-paced running.
   3. Running can be very effective in maintaining circulatory endurance.
   4. Aerobics—a total fitness program designed to improve cardiovascular endurance.

V. Circuit Training

A. A circuit is a number of carefully selected exercises which are arranged and numbered consecutively: the exercises range over a given area.

B. Circuit training increases muscular strength, muscular endurance, and cardiovascular endurance.

C. Planning a Circuit
   1. Your circuit depends on your aims.
   2. Exercises must be
      a. strenuous
      b. standardized
      c. balanced
   3. Circuit patterns can be designed to fit the needs of a group or individual.

VI. Rope Skipping

A. Rope skipping is an excellent cardiovascular exercise.

B. Ten minutes of rope skipping is as helpful in maintaining cardiovascular endurance as a 30-minute program of jogging.

VII. Sports

A. May serve as conditioning programs.

B. If a sport is to supply the requirements of a physical fitness program, it must be vigorous. A person should participate in it at least three sessions a week. Ideally, he should participate in it for 60 minutes every day.

VIII. Use of Leisure Time

A. Begin to spend your time in activities that will help to reacquaint you with the environment.

B. Protect the Environment.

QUESTIONS FOR REVIEW

1. Choose one of your problem areas, and use calisthenic exercises to improve this area.
2. What is the value of a calisthenic program?
3. Fill out a program card for yourself. Plan a weight training program that would improve your strength.
4. What three types of exercise are ideal for improving circulatory endurance?
5. How should a pregnant woman handle the problem of exercise during her pregnancy?
6. Follow a jogging program for one month. Check your resting pulse rate to determine whether it has dropped in the month. Why should this happen?
7. Take the Aerobics Fitness Test. How do you score? What condition are you in?

BIBLIOGRAPHY

Bowerman, William J., W. E. Harris, with James M. Shea, *Jogging*, New York, Grosset & Dunlap, 1967.

Brash, James C., ed., *D. J. Cunningham's Manual of Practical Anatomy*, 12th ed., New York, Oxford University Press, 1958.

Bullen, Beverly A., and C. C. Conrad, "Physical Fitness of Children and Adolescents," *CAHPER Journal*, Vol. 31, No. 5 (March/April, 1970), pp. 7–9, 34.

Buskirk, Elsworth R., and Joseph Brozek, "Unilateral Activity and Bone and Muscle Development in the Forearm," *Research Quarterly*, Vol. 27, No. 2 (May 1965), pp. 127–141.

Buskirk, Elsworth R., and J. E. Counsilman, *Science and Medicine of Exercise and Sports*, New York, Harper & Row, 1960.

Cooper, Kenneth L., *The New Aerobics*, New York, Bantam Books, 1970.

Davis, E. C., G. A. Logan, and W. C. McKinney, *Biophysical Values of Muscular Activity*, Dubuque, Iowa, Wm. C. Brown, 1965.

deVries, Herbert A., *Physiology of Exercise*, Dubuque, Iowa, Wm. C. Brown, 1966.

Dexter, Genevie, "The California Physical Performance Test," *CAHPER Journal*, Vol. 33, No. 4 (January/February, 1971), pp. 11, 18.

Grollman, Sigmund, *The Human Body*, 2nd ed., New York, The Macmillan Co., 1969.

Hairabedian, Ara, "Physical Fitness," *CAHPER Journal*, Vol. 34, No. 2 (September/October, 1971), pp. 6, 20.

Hardin, Garrett, *Biology, Its Principles and Implications*, 2nd ed., San Francisco, W. H. Freeman and Co., 1966.

Howell, M. L., and W. R. Morford, "Circuit Training," *Journal of Health, Physical Education and Recreation* (November 1961), Vol. 32, No. 8, p. 33.

Isola, Frank E., "Exercising for Physical Fitness," *CAHPER Journal*, Vol. 32, No. 3 (November/December, 1969), pp. 7, 28, 29.

Jacoby, Edward G., *Physiological Implications of Interval Training*. Idaho Falls, Idaho, Idaho Falls School District. Unpublished thesis.

Johnson, Harry J., "Jogging: Bad Jolt for the Heart?" *Medical World News*, Vol. 10, No. 36 (September 5, 1969), p. 32.

Kasch, F. W., "How Much Should I Exercise?" *California School Health*, Vol. 4, No. 4 (June, 1969), pp. 9–11.

Kinger, Diana Clifford, C. E. Gray, and C. E. Stackpole, *Anatomy and Physiology*, 15th ed., New York, The Macmillan Co., 1966.

Langley, L. L., E. Cheraskin, and R. Sleeper, *Dynamic Anatomy and Physiology*, 2nd ed., New York, McGraw-Hill, Inc., 1963.

Linde, Alexander R., "Isometrics: A No-No for the Flabby?" *Medical World News*, Vol. 11, No. 28 (July 10, 1970), p. 17.

Mayer, Jean, "Exercise and Weight Control," Chapter 12, *Exercise and Fitness* (A Collection of Papers Presented at the Colloquim on Exercise and Fitness), University of Illinois, Urbana, Illinois, 1960, pp. 110–121.

Memmler, Ruth Lundeed, *The Human Body in Health and Disease*, 2nd ed., Philadelphia, J. B. Lippincott Co., 1962.

Morgan, R. E. and G. T. Adamson, *Circuit Training*, 2nd ed., Bell & Sons, London, 1961.

Nason, Alvin, *Textbook of Modern Biology*, New York, John Wiley and Sons, Inc., 1965.

Ricci, Benjamin, *Physical and Physiological Conditioning for Men*, Dubuque, Iowa, Wm. C. Brown Co., 1966.

Royal Canadian Air Force Exercise Plan For Physical Fitness, New York, Simon and Schuster, Inc., 1962.

Scientific American, *The Living Cell*, San Francisco, W. H. Freeman and Co., 1965.

Stiles, Merritt H., "Names in the News," *Medical World News*, Vol. 12, No. 10 (March 12, 1971), p. 68.

Strand, Fleur L., *Modern Physiology: The Chemical and Structural Basis and Function*, New York, The Macmillan Co., 1965.

Swatek, Paul, *The User's Guide to the Protection of the Environment*, New York, Ballantine Books, 1970.

White, Paul D., "The Role of Exercise in the Aging," *Journal of the American Medical Association*, Vol. 165, No. 1 (1957), pp. 70–71.

Wilkenson, Bud, *Modern Physical Fitness*, New York, Barnes & Noble Inc., 1969.

Windle, Will F., *Textbooks of Histology*, 3rd ed., New York, McGraw-Hill, Inc., 1960.

Glossary

adduct	To draw toward the center or median line of the body.
aerobic	Metabolizing only in the presence of oxygen.
alveolus	A small cavity; an air sac which is terminal dilation of the bronchioles in the lungs.
anabolism	The building up of the body; constructive metabolism.
arteriosclerosis	A condition in which the arteries become thickened and hardened and lose their elasticity.

bursa	A closed sac lined with synovial membrane containing fluid, found over an exposed and prominent part of a bone.
calorie	A unit of heat. The large or kilocalorie (C) is the amount of heat required to raise 1 Kg. of water from 15° to 16° C.
carbohydrates	A group of compounds including the sugars and starches.
cartilage	The gristle or elastic substance attached at the joints of bones; or forming certain parts of the body (ear, nose, etc.).
catabolism	Destructive metabolism. Any destructive process by which complex substances are converted by living cells into more simple compounds.
cholesterol	A white, fatty, crystalline substance, tasteless and odorless, found in bile, blood, gallstones, egg yolk, and many other animal products.
configuration	The general form of the body.
defecation	The discharge of fecal material from the bowel.
fat	Whitish animal or plant substance. In humans it is stored in adipose tissue.
intramuscular	Within a muscle.
metabolism	The sum of all the physical and chemical processes of the body.
optimum	The best or most favorable point, degree, amount, condition, etc.
phlegm	Abnormally large amounts of viscous mucus discharged through the mouth.
protein	An organic compound consisting of a chain of many amino acids.
sedentary	Being inactive. Doing as little as possible, accustomed to very little exercise.
vascularization	The process of supplying tissue with blood vessels.

Index

Italic numbers refer to pages with illustrations; t = table